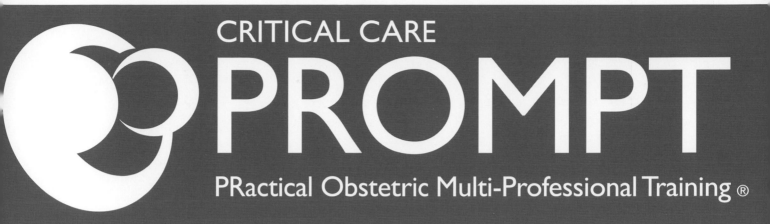

CRITICAL CARE
PROMPT
PRactical Obstetric Multi-Professional Training ®

PROMPT CiPP

Care of the Critically ill Pregnant or Postpartum woman

Course Handbook

Edited by

The PROMPT Editorial Team

CAMBRIDGE
UNIVERSITY PRESS

University Printing House, Cambridge CB2 8BS, United Kingdom

One Liberty Plaza, 20th Floor, New York, NY 10006, USA

477 Williamstown Road, Port Melbourne, VIC 3207, Australia

314–321, 3rd Floor, Plot 3, Splendor Forum, Jasola District Centre, New Delhi – 110025, India

79 Anson Road, #06-04/06, Singapore 079906

Cambridge University Press is part of the University of Cambridge.

It furthers the University's mission by disseminating knowledge in the pursuit of education, learning, and research at the highest international levels of excellence.

www.cambridge.org
Information on this title: www.cambridge.org/9781108433167
DOI: 10.1017/9781108377348
© 2019 PROMPT Maternity Foundation

Registered Charity in England and Wales No. 1140557
Registered Company No. 7506593
Registered Office: Stone King LLP, 13 Queen Square, Bath, BA1 2HJ
www.promptmaternity.org

First published 2019
Reprinted 2019

Printed in Singapore by Markono Print Media Pte Ltd

A catalogue record for this publication is available from the British Library.

ISBN 978-1-108-43316-7 Paperback

Every effort has been made in preparing this book to provide accurate and up-to-date information that is in accord with accepted standards and practice at the time of publication. Although case histories are drawn from actual cases, every effort has been made to disguise the identities of the individuals involved. Nevertheless, the authors, editors, and publishers can make no warranties that the information contained herein is totally free from error, not least because clinical standards are constantly changing through research and regulation. The authors, editors, and publishers therefore disclaim all liability for direct or consequential damages resulting from the use of material contained in this book. Readers are strongly advised to pay careful attention to information provided by the manufacturer of any drugs or equipment that they plan to use.

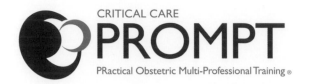

CRITICAL CARE
PROMPT
PRactical Obstetric Multi-Professional Training ®

IMPORTANT GUIDANCE FOR USERS of the PROMPT CIPP (Care of the Critically ill Pregnant or Postpartum woman) Course Handbook

Every reasonable effort has been made in preparing this Prompt CiPP Course Handbook to provide accurate and up-to-date information which is in accord with accepted standards and practice. Nevertheless, the authors and editors can make no warranties that the information contained herein is totally free from inaccuracy or error, not least because clinical standards are constantly changing through research and regulation. The authors and editors therefore disclaim (to the fullest extent possible under English law) all liability for all direct and/or consequential damages resulting from the use of any material contained within this handbook and the reader is irrevocably deemed to accept and agree with the authors and editors' absence of liability and culpability.

The PROMPT CiPP Course Handbook was developed for attendees of the PROMPT CiPP Course, a Maternal Critical Care training course that is a constituent part of the third edition PROMPT 'Course in a Box'.

The PROMPT Maternity Foundation (PMF) is a multi-professional group of obstetricians, gynaecologists, midwives and anaesthetists. PMF is a company limited by guarantee (Company Number 7506593) and is registered as a charity with the Charity Commission for England & Wales (Charity Number 1140557). PMF has experience in providing materials and tools for multi-professional obstetric emergencies training. For further information visit: https://www.promptmaternity.org

September 2018

Contents

Editorial team & contributors   4

Acknowledgements   5

List of abbreviations and terms   6

Section 1: Introduction to Maternal Critical Care   9

Section 2: Recognition of the critically ill pregnant or postpartum woman   20

Section 3: Structured approach to the review of a critically ill pregnant or postpartum woman   31

Section 4: Oxygen administration and blood gas interpretation   51

Section 5: ECGs and rhythm recognition   60

Section 6: Invasive monitoring   79

Section 7: Cardio-respiratory emergencies in pregnant and postpartum women   92

Section 8: Neurological emergencies in pregnant and postpartum women   110

Section 9: Sepsis and the critically ill pregnant or postpartum woman   122

Editorial Team and Contributors

PROMPT Editorial Team

Jane Ashby-Styles	Senior Anaesthetic Nurse, Bristol
Jo Crofts	Consultant Obstetrician, Bristol
Chris Laxton	Consultant Anaesthetist, Bristol
Neil Muchatuta	Consultant Anaesthetist, Bristol
Karine Zander	CiPP Course Director & Consultant Anaesthetist, Bristol

Contributors

Fiona Donald	Consultant Anaesthetist, Bristol
Matthew Martin	Specialist Registrar in Intensive Care Medicine and Anaesthesia, Bristol
Kate O'Connor	Consultant Anaesthetist, Bristol
Andrew Ray	Specialist Registrar in Intensive Care Medicine and Anaesthesia, Bristol
Reston Smith	Consultant Anaesthetist and Intensivist, Bristol
Cathy Winter	Senior Midwife, Bristol
Elaine Yard	Senior Midwife, Bristol

Acknowledgements

Thank you to all the maternity staff at North Bristol NHS Trust for their valuable contributions to this maternal critical care course handbook.

List of abbreviations & terms

ABCDE	Airway, Breathing, Circulation, Disability, Exposure
ABG	Arterial blood gas
ADH	Antidiuretic hormone
AF	Atrial fibrillation
ALS	Advanced life support
ARF	Acute renal failure
AV node	Atrioventricular node
AVPU	Alert, responds to Voice, responds to Painful stimuli, Unresponsive
BiPAP	Bi-level positive airway pressure
BP	Blood pressure
bpm	Beats per minute
CiPP	Care of the Critically ill Pregnant or Postpartum woman
CO_2	Carbon dioxide
COPD	Chronic obstructive pulmonary disease
CPAP	Continuous positive airway pressure
CPP	Cerebral perfusion pressure
CPR	Cardiopulmonary resuscitation
CRP	C-reactive protein
CT	Computed tomography
CTPA	CT pulmonary angiogram
CVE	Cerebrovascular event
CVP	Central venous pressure
CVS	Chorionic villous sampling
CXR	Chest x-ray
DIC	Disseminated intravascular coagulation
DVT	Deep vein thrombosis
Echo	Echocardiogram
ECMO	Extracorporeal membrane oxygenation

ECG	Electrocardiograph
FBC	Full blood count
FiO_2	Fraction of inspired oxygen
G&S	Group and save (also known as group and screen)
GCS	Glasgow coma scale
GI	Gastrointestinal
GP	General practitioner
H_2-receptors	Histamine-2 receptors
HCO_3^-	Bicarbonate
HELLP	Haemolysis, elevated liver enzymes and low platelets
HR	Heart rate
ICP	Intracranial pressure
ICU	Intensive care unit
IUGR	Intrauterine growth restriction
IM	Intramuscular
IV	Intravenous
IVC	Inferior vena cava
LFTs	Liver function tests
LMWH	Low-molecular-weight heparin
MAP	Mean arterial pressure
MBRRACE-UK	Mothers and Babies: Reducing Risk through Audits and Confidential Enquires across the UK
MCC	Maternal Critical Care
M,C & S	Microscopy, culture and sensitivity
$MgSO_4$	Magnesium Sulfate
MI	Myocardial infarction
MOEWS	Modified obstetric early warning scoring systems
MRI	Magnetic resonance imaging
NaCl	Sodium chloride
NG	Nasogastric
NSAID	Non-steroidal anti-inflammatory drug

NSTEMI	Non-ST-elevation myocardial infarction
O_2	Oxygen
$PaCO_2$	Arterial partial pressure of carbon dioxide
PaO_2	Arterial partial pressure of oxygen
PCI	Percutaneous coronary intervention
PE	Pulmonary embolus
PEA	Pulseless electrical activity
PEFR	Peak expiratory flow rate
PERLA	Pupils equal and reactive to light and accommodation
PET	Pre-eclamptic toxaemia
PPI	Proton pump inhibitor
PR	Per rectum
PTSD	Post-traumatic stress disorder
RR	Respiratory rate
SC	Subcutaneous
$ScvO_2$	Central venous saturation of oxygen
SA node	Sinoatrial node
SGA	Small for gestational age
SIADH	Syndrome of inappropriate antidiuretic hormone secretion
SOB	Short of breath
SpO_2	Peripheral saturation of oxygen
STEMI	ST-elevation myocardial infarction
SVC	Superior vena cava
TPN	Total parental nutrition
U&E	Urea and electrolytes
VBG	Venous blood gas
V/Q	Ventilation/perfusion
VF	Ventricular fibrillation
VT	Ventricular tachycardia
VTE	Venous thromboembolism

Section 1: Introduction to Maternal Critical Care

Key Learning Points

- Maternal critical care is required for pregnant and postnatal women with complex medical and obstetric problems
- There should be appropriate critical care support to manage pregnant and postpartum women who become unwell and this should be provided on the labour ward or a maternal critical care unit
- Maternal critical care requires a multi-professional team of midwives, obstetricians, neonatologists (if mother still pregnant), anaesthetists and intensive care specialists
- Specialised maternal critical care charts should be used to document observations, fluid balance, ongoing clinical investigations, results and medical reviews
- Maternal critical care worksheets provide a useful framework for structured medical review
- Women requiring critical care should receive frequent obstetric reviews to ensure the maintenance of their usual antenatal and postnatal maternity care
- All health care professionals should be aware of the potential long-term effects of a 'near-miss' incident on a mother's health, in particular their mental health

Introduction

Maternal Critical Care is the specialised care of pregnant or postpartum women whose conditions are life-threatening and require comprehensive care and close monitoring. In the UK, and in many countries worldwide, pregnancy care is increasingly complex as the pregnant population becomes older, more obese and has more medical co-morbidities (1). Due to these changing demographics, women are more likely to experience pregnancy-related complications that may require critical care. Women aged 35 and over have a significantly higher maternal mortality rate than women aged 20–24, with 84% of maternal deaths in the UK between 2009 and 2012 having multiple medical co-morbidities and/or significant social factors (1).

In Europe between one and three women for every 1,000 births are admitted to an intensive care unit (ICU) (2). In the USA it is estimated that up to eight women per 1,000 births are admitted to an ICU (3). Most admissions to an ICU are made in the immediate postnatal period, with the most common reasons for admission including postpartum haemorrhage, complications of pre-eclampsia and hypertension, sepsis and cardiac disease (2).

The RCOG report *'Providing equity of critical and maternity care for the critically ill pregnant or recently pregnant woman'* released in 2011, stated that: "Childbirth is a major life event for women and their families. The few women who become critically ill during this time should receive the same standard of care for both their pregnancy-related and critical care needs, delivered by professionals with the same competency levels irrespective of whether these are provided in a maternity or general critical care setting." (4). Furthermore, the MBRRACE-UK *'Saving Lives, Improving Mothers' Care'* (2014) report also recommended: **"**There should be adequate provision of appropriate critical care support for the management of a pregnant woman who becomes unwell. Plans should be in place for the provision of critical care on labour wards or maternity care on critical care units, depending on the most appropriate setting for a pregnant or postpartum woman to receive care" (1).

In August 2018, the Royal College of Anaesthetists (RCoA) released an updated Report *'Care of the critically ill woman in childbirth; enhanced maternal care.'* (5). The document has been produced by a joint working party comprising of representatives from; Obstetric Anaesthetists Association (OAA), Royal College of Anaesthetists (RCoA), Royal College of Midwives (RCM), Royal College of Obstetricians and Gynaecologists (RCOG), Intensive Care Society and The Faculty of Intensive Care Medicine. The report identifies the urgent need for teamwork and multi-disciplinary training in the early recognition of critical illness and also includes reflections from two women who became critically ill peri-partum, emphasising the importance of the woman's voice too.

The report recognises that many of the recommendations from the 2011 RCOG Report have not yet been implemented in UK maternity units, and therefore requests that there should be a nationwide implementation of the recommendations contained within the 2018 report. The key messages for enhanced maternal care (EMC) in the 2018 report include:

- Working in teams is vital for good outcomes
- Training for enhanced maternal care should be competency-based
- ***Multi-professional education and training is essential***
- There is a need for a national early warning system modified for obstetrics (MOEWS)
- Whilst care should usually take place on the labour ward, transfer to ITU may occasionally be warranted
- Women admitted to general ITU should receive coordinated shared care and daily multi-professional reviews

The recommendations for education and training are in line with the content of this PROMPT CiPP training package, with emphasis upon multi-disciplinary team training and simulation-based learning techniques. The 2018 Report also includes the *'Enhanced Maternal Care competency framework for midwives caring for the ill and acutely ill woman'* which is produced by the RCM in collaboration with the OAA.

Why is 'maternal' critical care different from 'normal' critical care?

The provision of critical care for women who are pregnant or who have recently given birth provides different challenges to those of the general adult population.

- The pregnant, critically ill, woman requires monitoring and multi-professional management, as does her unborn child. Such care will require the combined knowledge and skills of midwives, obstetricians, anaesthetists and intensive care specialists. When an urgent birth is necessary because of deterioration in the woman's condition, there is a need for immediate access to an operating theatre, neonatal resuscitation facilities and the neonatal unit.

- There is often no ideal location to provide critical care for pregnant women: giving birth in the intensive care unit (ICU) is not ideal as ICU staff may not have the skills to deal with obstetric complications, whereas labour wards often do not have the facilities to provide invasive ventilation or to support women with multi-organ failure. The overriding principle is that a pregnant woman must receive the correct level of care wherever she is. Maternal critical care is most commonly provided in an adequately-equipped and staffed labour ward for antenatal and intrapartum care but transfer to a General ICU may be required if there is further deterioration in the mother's clinical condition.

- The physiological changes of pregnancy provide an increased physiological reserve however they also impose increased physiological demands.

  o The airway can be more difficult to intubate if invasive ventilation is required.

  o There is an increased oxygen demand and reduced oxygen reserve with reduced lung compliance. This means hypoxia is more likely and adequate ventilation can be harder to achieve (6).

  o Aortocaval compression must be considered after 20 weeks' gestation.

  o Cardiac output increases significantly during pregnancy.

  o Not all medications can be safely given in pregnancy, and those that can, may have altered plasma levels.

- o The immunosuppression associated with pregnancy means that infection and sepsis can be more common, more aggressive and may be due to atypical organisms.

- o Regurgitation and aspiration of gastric contents and venous thromboembolism (VTE) are more common; prophylaxis should be considered for these potential complications.

- The critically ill woman who has recently given birth should, if possible, have continued contact with her baby to support the establishment of breastfeeding and bonding (7). Such contact can often be achieved in a maternity unit but is more difficult to achieve in an ICU. Separation of mother and baby can lead to maternal emotional distress, which may inhibit the establishment of breastfeeding and increase the risk of postnatal depression.

- Caring for mother and baby in separate locations can also be stressful for the family who are forced to divide their time between the unwell mother and her newborn baby. Care should be as holistic as possible, without compromising clinical practice.

When might maternal critical care be required?

There are multiple conditions where a pregnant woman, or woman who has recently given birth, may require critical care. No list will ever be comprehensive but common conditions may include those listed in **Table 1.1**.

Table 1.1 Possible conditions requiring maternal critical care

Possible conditions requiring maternal critical care	
Respiratory	▪ Severe community acquired pneumonia (including influenza) ▪ Pulmonary oedema ▪ Severe asthma ▪ Pulmonary embolism ▪ Bronchospasm
Cardiovascular	▪ Severe uncontrolled hypertension ▪ Cardiomyopathy ▪ Massive haemorrhage ▪ Pulmonary embolism ▪ Septic shock
Sepsis	▪ Obstetric related: e.g. chorioamnionitis, post-operative, mastitis, UTI ▪ Non-obstetric: influenza, pneumonia, meningitis
Neurological	▪ Status epilepticus ▪ Meningitis ▪ Intracerebral bleed ▪ Malignancy ▪ Guillain-Barré syndrome

Recognition of the critically ill pregnant or postpartum woman

Early detection of mothers who may require critical care can be challenging. Severe illness in pregnancy is relatively rare and the normal physiological changes that occur with pregnancy can mask the early warning signs normally seen in a clinically deteriorating woman. Breathlessness is a common feature of pregnancy, however persistent breathlessness when lying flat needs investigating as it may be due to undiagnosed cardiac disease (8).

> As highlighted in a recently published MBRRACE-UK report, reduced or altered conscious level is not an early warning sign; it is a red flag to indicate established illness, and should be acted on immediately and appropriately (8).

Mothers who report feeling unwell, who look unwell, and/or report a 'feeling that something awful is going to happen' should be thoroughly assessed. It is not always necessary to wait until observations deteriorate: early recognition of critical illness, prompt involvement of senior clinical staff and multi-professional involvement save lives and remain the key factors for high-quality care for sick mothers (8). More information on the use of modified obstetric early warning scoring systems (MOEWS) and Maternity Critical Care Charts can be found in **Section 2.**

Investigations for critically ill pregnant and postpartum women

Most investigations can be carried out safely in pregnancy without risk to the mother or the fetus. Investigations to diagnose or exclude life-threatening conditions should therefore not be denied or delayed. Where uncertainty about the safety of an investigation exists, a multi-professional discussion between senior obstetric and radiology clinicians can be helpful in determining the most appropriate and safe way to proceed.

> **'Women should not be denied relevant investigations or treatments for life-threatening conditions, simply because they are pregnant or breastfeeding.'**
>
> MBRRACE-UK 2016 (7).

Where should maternal critical care be provided?

Currently, most maternal critical care is provided within intensive care units (ICU), however critical care should be a *level* of care provision, rather than a *location*. Most aspects of maternal critical care can be provided outside the ICU, including on the labour ward or obstetric theatres.

Women who require advanced respiratory or prolonged cardiovascular support will usually require transfer to an ICU for invasive monitoring and specialised care. Respiratory support may require mechanical ventilation, whilst cardiovascular support may include use of inotropes (medications that increase the force of contraction of the heart to increase cardiac output and blood flow to vital organs) or vasopressors (medications that constrict arteries to increase mean arterial pressure and therefore organ perfusion). However, women requiring Level 2 critical care (see **Table 1.2**) may be able to remain within the maternity unit if trained staff and suitable monitoring equipment are available. If feasible, critical care services should be brought to the woman rather than changing her location (1).

The Intensive Care Society's *Levels of Critical Care Support for Adult Patients* classification of critical care focuses on the level of dependency that individual patients need and the appropriate location for the provision of this level of care, and is now implemented in most NHS institutions (9). Examples of different levels of care that may be required in maternity are listed in **Table 1.2**.

Table 1.2 Levels of critical care, with examples from maternal critical care (4)

Level of care	Definition	Maternity Example
Level 0	Women whose needs can be met through normal ward care in an acute hospital	Care of a low risk mother
Level 1	Women at risk of their condition deteriorating, or those recently relocated from higher levels of care, whose needs can be met on an acute ward with additional advice and support from the Critical Care team	▪ Risk of haemorrhage ▪ Oxytocin infusion ▪ Mild pre-eclampsia on oral anti-hypertensives/fluid restriction ▪ Woman with medical condition, e.g. congenital heart disease, diabetes requiring sliding scale insulin
Level 2	Women requiring more detailed observation or intervention including support for a single failing organ system or post-operative care and those 'stepping down' from higher levels of care	Basic Respiratory Support ▪ 50% or more oxygen via facemask to maintain oxygen saturation ▪ Continuous positive airway pressure (CPAP) ▪ Bi-level positive airway pressure (BIPAP) Basic Cardiovascular Support ▪ Intravenous anti-hypertensives to control blood pressure ▪ Arterial line for pressure monitoring or sampling ▪ CVP line for fluid management and CVP monitoring to guide therapy Advanced Cardiovascular Support ▪ Simultaneous use of at least two intravenous, anti-arrhythmic/anti-hypertensive/vasoactive drugs, one of which must be a vasoactive drug ▪ Need to measure and treat cardiac output Neurological Support ▪ Magnesium infusion to control seizures (not prophylaxis) ▪ Intracranial pressure monitoring Hepatic support ▪ Management of acute fulminant hepatic failure, e.g. from HELLP syndrome or acute fatty liver, such that transplantation is being considered
Level 3	Women requiring advanced respiratory support alone, or basic respiratory support together with support of at least two organ systems. This level includes all women requiring support for multi-organ failure.	Advanced Respiratory Support ▪ Invasive mechanical ventilation (i.e. intubation and ventilation) Support of two or more organ systems ▪ Renal support plus Basic Respiratory Support ▪ Basic Respiratory/Cardiovascular Support plus an additional organ supported

Regular structured review: ongoing assessment and management

All women receiving critical care require a comprehensive, structured and regular medical review for early detection of problems and timely interventions. A systematic approach should be employed using a standard ABCDE approach, together with review of medications, venous thromboembolism prophylaxis, kidney and bowel function, pain management, fluid balance and nutritional assessment. More information on the structured review of the critically ill pregnant or postpartum woman and use of a Maternal Critical Care Chart is provided in **Sections 2 and 3**.

Equipment required

The RCOG's Maternal Critical Care Working Group have produced guidance on the minimum equipment required for the provision of Maternity Critical Care (4). This is listed in **Figure 1.1** below.

Figure 1.1 Minimum equipment list for provision of maternal critical care (4)

Minimum equipment list for provision of maternal critical care* (RCOG 2011)
▪ Monitor for HR, BP, ECG, SpO_2 and transducer for invasive monitoring
▪ Piped oxygen and suction
▪ Intravenous fluid warmer
▪ Forced air warming device
▪ Blood gas analyser
▪ Infusion pumps
▪ Emergency massive haemorrhage trolley
▪ Emergency eclampsia box
▪ Transfer equipment – monitor and ventilator
▪ Computer terminal to facilitate access to blood results, PACS system
▪ Copy of hospital obstetric guidelines including Maternal Critical Care
▪ Resuscitation trolley with defibrillator and airway management equipment
* Many of these items may already be available in maternity theatres or on the labour ward

Transfer of the critically ill pregnant or postpartum woman to Intensive Care

Critically ill pregnant or postpartum women may need transferred from the labour ward to other locations including the ICU radiology, operating theatres or another hospital. All transfers risk destabilisation and deterioration and therefore require specialised equipment and personnel. Transfers should be timely, coordinated and well-planned so they can be safely accomplished (1).

Senior doctors should assess the woman and engage in multi-professional discussion to determine the best location for on-going care. Once a decision is made there should be one single transfer to definitive care. Decisions must include the means and timing of intra- or inter-hospital transfer to ensure that the transfer is carried out safely (10).

Transfers should not be undertaken until the woman has been resuscitated and stabilised. In many circumstances an 'ICU outreach team' will attend to assist with both preparation and transfer.

- Before transfer to the ICU it may be necessary to secure the woman's airway with an endotracheal tube (with appropriate end-tidal carbon dioxide monitoring), rather than risk deterioration *en route*.

- Appropriate intravenous access must be in place.

- Continuous invasive blood pressure measurement is the best technique for monitoring blood pressure during the transfer of ill women and therefore an arterial line may need to be sited before transfer.

- Adequate supplies of oxygen, intravenous fluids, resuscitation drugs and blood products (if required) must be available prior to transfer.

If a woman is transferred to an ICU for ongoing management there should be a daily consultant obstetric and midwifery review, even if only in a supportive role, until such time that the woman can be repatriated to the maternity unit. Regular information and neonatal updates, including photos of their baby, can be very helpful.

Longer-term impacts of near-miss maternal morbidity for women, their babies and families

Women should be aware that their experience of a 'near-miss' incident can have long-lasting effects on their health, particularly their mental health, and may also affect their partner (11). Research suggests that one in five ICU survivors have developed a post-traumatic stress disorder (PTSD) at one year following discharge (12). Follow-up consultations can be helpful and may reduce symptoms of post-traumatic stress at 3 to 6 months after ICU discharge (13).

The 2018 RCoA Report includes 2 vignettes of women's reflections after experiencing critical illness, and they both provide excellent accounts of the impact of their illness on both them, and their families (5).

Community midwives and GPs should be informed when a woman is discharged from hospital after an episode of critical care. Follow-up appointments with the obstetrician and/or midwifery staff can be helpful and should be arranged for at least six weeks postnatally or sometimes longer afterwards, depending on the mother's recovery and also the collation of any test results that may be necessary for the follow-up appointment.

References

1.   Knight M, Kenyon S, Brocklehurst P, Neilson J, Shakespeare J, Kurinczuk JJ, on behalf of MBRACCE-UK. Saving Lives, Improving Mothers' Care. Oxford National Perinatal Epidemiology Unit, University of Oxford. 2014.

2.   Zwart JJ, Dupuis JRO, Richters A, Öry F, van Roosmalen J. Obstetric intensive care unit admission: a 2-year nationwide population-based cohort study. Intensive Care Med. 2009 Nov 10;36(2):256–63.

3.   ACOG Practice Bulletin No. 100: Critical care in pregnancy. Obstetrics & Gynecology. 2009 Feb;113(2 Pt 1):443–50.

4.   RCOG. Providing equity of critical and maternity care for the critically ill pregnant or recently pregnant woman. 2011 Jul 13:1–58. https://www.rcog.org.uk/globalassets/documents/guidelines/prov_eq_matandcritcare.pdf. Accessed December 2nd 2017.

5.   Royal College of Anaesthetists. Care of the critically ill woman in childbirth; enhanced maternal care 2018. August 2018

6.   Truhlář A, Deakin CD, Soar J, Khalifa GEA, Alfonzo A, Bierens JJLM, et al. European Resuscitation Council Guidelines for Resuscitation 2015: Section 4. Cardiac arrest in special circumstances. Resuscitation. European Resuscitation Council, American Heart Association, Inc., and International Liaison Committee on Resuscitation. Published by Elsevier Ireland Ltd; 2015 Oct 1;95:148–201.

7.   RCOG. Minimum Standards for the Organisation and Delivery of Care in Labour. 2007 Oct 8:1–89. https://www.rcog.org.uk/globalassets/documents/guidelines/wprsaferchildbirthreport2007.pdf. Accessed 2nd December 2017.

8.   Knight M, Nair M, Tuffnell D, Kenyon S, Shakespeare J, Brocklehurst P, et al. Saving Lives, Improving Mothers' Care. Knight M, Nair M, Tuffnell D, Kenyon S, Shakespeare J, Brocklehurst P, on behalf of MBRRACE-UK. Oxford National Perinatal Epidemiology Unit, University of Oxford. 2016.

9.   Intensive Care Society. Levels of Critical Care for Adult Patients. 2010 Jan 14:1–12. https://www.ics.ac.uk/AsiCommon/Controls/BSA/Downloader.aspx?iDocumentStorageKey=2a465b42-21e3-499b-a955-fe72f844dd70&iFileTypeCode=PDF&iFileName=Unlicenced%20Medicines%20in%20Intensive%20Care. Accessed 2nd December 2017.

10.   AAGBI. Interhospital Transfer. 2009 Jan 29:1–20. Available from https://www.aagbi.org/sites/default/files/interhospital09.pdf. Accessed 2nd December 2017.

11.   Knight M, Acosta C, Brocklehurst P, Cheshire A, Fitzpatrick K, Hinton L, et al. Beyond maternal death: improving the quality of maternal care through national studies of "near-miss" maternal morbidity. Southampton (UK): NIHR Journals Library; 2016. https://www.ncbi.nlm.nih.gov/books/NBK368642/pdf/Bookshelf_NBK368642.pdf. Accessed 2nd December 2017.

12.   Parker AM, Sricharoenchai T, Raparla S, Schneck KW, Bienvenu OJ, Needham DM. Posttraumatic stress disorder in critical illness survivors: a meta-analysis. Critical Care Medicine. 2015 May;43(5):1121–9.

13.   Jensen JF, Thomsen T, Overgaard D, Bestle MH, Christensen D, Egerod I. Impact of follow-up consultations for ICU survivors on post-ICU syndrome: a systematic review and meta-analysis. Intensive Care Med. 2015 May;41(5):763–75.

Further reading

Competencies for Recognising and Responding to Acutely Ill Patients in Hospital. DH, London 2008
www.dh.gov.uk/en/Publicationsandstatistics/Publications/PublicationsPolicyAndGuidance/DH_096989

Intercollegiate Maternal Critical Care (MCC) Sub-Committee of the Obstetric Anaesthetist Association:
Maternity Enhanced Care Competencies Required by Midwives Caring for Acutely Ill Women. 2015

www.oaa-anes.ac.uk/assets/_managed/cms/files/MEC%20May%202015%20v13-03.pdf

Notes:

Section 2: Recognition of the critically ill pregnant or postpartum woman

---

Key learning points

Recognition of the deteriorating critically ill pregnant or postpartum woman:

- Modified obstetric early warning scoring systems (MOEWS)
- Initial assessment and immediate management

On-going care of a deteriorating critically ill woman:

- Place of care
- Regular structured review
- Use of dedicated 'critical care' charts to facilitate timely intervention and optimise on-going management

Recognition of the deteriorating critically ill pregnant or postpartum woman

Early detection of severely ill mothers can be challenging. Severe illness in pregnancy is relatively rare and the normal physiological changes of pregnancy can mask the early warning signs normally seen in a deteriorating non-pregnant woman. A good early warning sign of deterioration in pregnancy is that the woman looks unwell. She may become agitated, say she feels unwell or that she has a 'bad feeling about herself'. If you suspect the woman is deteriorating or she feels unwell (even if there is no change in the woman's observations) this should immediately be reported. Do not wait until the observations change – early recognition and early treatment saves lives.

Modified obstetric early warning scoring systems (MOEWS)

The modified obstetric early warning scoring system (MOEWS) combines physiological parameters with a scoring system to facilitate early recognition of, and intervention in, deteriorating pregnant or postpartum women. However, be aware that physiological changes of pregnancy mean that women can mask and compensate for severe degrees of illness. Therefore, clinical judgment combined with a detailed history and examination are at least as important as completing, and acting upon, the MOEWS chart.

A MOEWS chart (**Figure 2.1**) should be used when plotting any maternal observations, except in labour when all observations should be plotted on the partogram (which should ideally include the same parameters as the MOEWS chart for the maternal observations section). Once critical care is indicated, a maternal critical care chart should be used (see **Figure 2.4**).

Figure 2.1 MOEWS chart and guidance

PROMPT - MODIFIED OBSTETRIC EARLY WARNING SCORE CHART
(FOR MATERNITY USE ONLY)

Frequency of observations

DATE	TIME	FREQUENCY (IN HRS)	SIGNED	PRINT	STATUS

Use identification label or :-
Name:
DOB:
Hospital No:

Ward:

	Date :																	
	Time :																	
Respirations (write rate in corresp. box)	>30																	>30
	21-30																	21-30
	11-20																	11-20
	0-10																	0-10
Saturations if applicable (write sats in corresp. box)	95-100%																	95-100%
	<95%																	<95%
Administered O_2 (L/min.)																		(L/min)
Temp	39																	39
	38																	38
	37																	37
	36																	36
	35																	35
Heart rate	170																	170
	160																	160
	150																	150
	140																	140
	130																	130
	120																	120
	110																	110
	100																	100
	90																	90
	80																	80
	70																	70
	60																	60
	50																	50
	40																	40
Systolic blood pressure	200																	200
	190																	190
	180																	180
	170																	170
	160																	160
	150																	150
	140																	140
	130																	130
	120																	120
	110																	110
	100																	100
	90																	90
	80																	80
	70																	70
	60																	60
	50																	50
Diastolic blood pressure	130																	130
	120																	120
	110																	110
	100																	100
	90																	90
	80																	80
	70																	70
	60																	60
	50																	50
	40																	40
Urine	passed (Y/N)																	passed (Y/N)
Proteinuria	protein ++																	protein ++
	protein >++																	protein >++
Amniotic fluid	Clear (C) Pink (P)																	Clear (C) Pink (P)
	Green (G)																	Green (G)
Neuro response (√)	Alert																	Alert
	Voice																	Voice
	Pain																	Pain
	Unresponsive																	Unresponsive
Pain Score (no.)	0-1																	0-1
	2-3																	2-3
Lochia	Normal (N)																	Normal (N)
	Heavy (H) Fresh (F) Offensive (O)																	Heavy(H) Fresh(F) Offensive (O)
Looks unwell	NO (√)																	NO (√)
	YES (√)																	YES (√)
Total Amber Scores																		
Total Red Scores																		

CONTACT DOCTOR FOR EARLY INTERVENTION IF WOMAN TRIGGERS ONE RED OR TWO AMBER SCORES AT ANY ONE TIME

FREQUENCY OF OBSERVATIONS This should be decided when the doctor or midwife commences the woman's chart. The frequency should be reviewed whenever there is a change in the woman's clinical condition and should be documented on the chart.

RESPIRATORY RATE: This is the single most important parameter for early detection of deterioration and should be measured at all monitoring events.

OXYGEN SATURATION: The level of administered oxygen (L/min) or 'air' should be documented with SpO_2. Oxygen should be prescribed on the drug chart.

TEMPERATURE: Temperature change may not necessarily be an effective measure of deterioration. A temperature rise or fall (> 37.5°C or < 36.0°C) may indicate sepsis. Sepsis can be difficult to recognise; if in doubt perform a venous or arterial blood gas to check pH and lactate and consult the Maternal Sepsis Risk Assessment tool.

HEART RATE: Another key sign – tachycardia may be the only sign of deterioration at an early stage. A tachycardic woman should be considered hypovolaemic until proven otherwise.

BLOOD PRESSURE: The physiological changes caused by pregnancy and childbirth can mean that early signs of impending collapse are not easily recognised.
Hypotension: this is a late sign of deterioration as it signifies decompensation and should be taken very seriously.
Hypertension: ALL pregnant women with a systolic blood pressure of 160 mm/Hg or higher must be treated (MBRRACE-UK 2016).

URINE OUTPUT: Urine output is one of the few signs of end-organ perfusion. This chart only identifies if urine is passed or not. Where indicated, a fluid balance chart should be used to document urine volume voided in millilitres.

NEUROLOGICAL RESPONSE: AVPU is a measure of the woman's level of consciousness. The best descriptor should be recorded. A change in conscious level should always be considered significant. A score of P or below is equivalent to Glasgow coma score of ≤ 8.
ALERT: fully awake woman
VOICE: drowsy but answers to name or some kind of response when addressed
PAIN: difficult to rouse, makes a response to sternal rubbing, pinching earlobes or shaking shoulders
UNRESPONSIVE: no response to voice, pain or other stimulus

TRUST YOUR INSTINCT

ADDITIONAL TOP TIPS
o   Do not be influenced by a previous record.
o   Do not look at the previous record until the new measurements have been taken.
o   If unsure or your readings do not seem correct, then repeat the readings.
o   High and low values are relevant e.g. BP and temperature.
o   If you cannot get an accurate recording, use manual techniques e.g. take the pulse rate manually, use a sphygmomanometer.
o   Never leave a value blank e.g. if you can't record a BP then write "unrecordable" and seek immediate help.

REMEMBER
REGULAR AND ACCURATE OBSERVATIONS ARE ESSENTIAL TO ALLOW EARLY RECOGNITON OF DETERIORATION.
ABNORMAL SCORES MUST TRIGGER AN APPROPRIATE RESPONSE. PASS ON THE INFORMATION AND PREPARE TO START TREATMENT.

PAIN SCORE: Pain scores guide analgesia and adequacy. They should be recorded as:
0   No pain
1   Mild pain
2   Moderate pain
3   Severe pain

Initial assessment and immediate management of a deteriorating pregnant or postpartum woman

The ABCDE approach

An ABCDE approach will enable the early detection of the most life-threatening problems and prompt the initiation of immediate treatment. When performing the initial assessment (primary survey) of a critically ill pregnant or postpartum woman (**Figure 2.2**), assessment <u>and</u> actions are typically completed for each system before moving onto the next (e.g. the airway needs to be opened before moving onto 'breathing'). Once the primary survey is complete, and any immediate interventions performed, a comprehensive structured review (**Figure 2.3**) should follow.

REMEMBER

**Early recognition and early treatment saves lives.
If in doubt, do not wait – call for help.**

**Dial 2222 in a peri-arrest / arrest situation:
survival is significantly worse if cardiac arrest occurs
(17–20% versus 40–45% if there is intervention before cardiac arrest)**

Place of care

The critically ill pregnant woman requires monitoring and multi-professional management, as does her unborn child. Such critical care requires the knowledge and skills of midwives, obstetricians, anaesthetists and intensive care specialists.

Women requiring advanced respiratory support (e.g. mechanical ventilation) or prolonged cardiovascular support with inotropes (medicines that increase the force of contraction of the heart to increase the cardiac output and maintain flow to vital organs and tissues) or vasopressors (drugs that increase the mean arterial pressure through arterial vasoconstriction) will require transfer to an ICU for intensive monitoring and specialised care.

However, women requiring Level 1 or 2 critical care may be able to remain within the maternity unit if trained staff and suitable monitoring equipment are available.

Figure 2.2 The Primary Survey: initial assessment and management of a deteriorating critically ill pregnant or postpartum woman

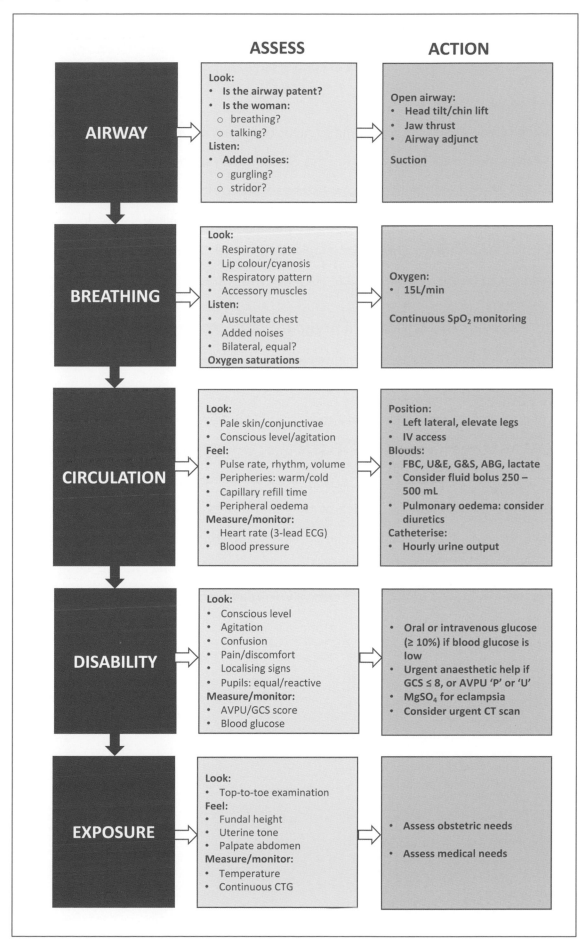

Examples of Level 2 care involving basic cardiovascular support include:

- o Arterial line for blood pressure monitoring or sampling
- o CVP line for fluid management
- o Intravenous anti-hypertensives to control blood pressure in pre-eclampsia

Key principles apply:

- o Midwives with sufficient training to meet necessary critical care competencies should be allocated to the woman as soon as possible with support from the midwifery team. Multi-professional input from anaesthetists and obstetricians is essential in all stages of care, with a minimum of four hourly assessment and review.
- o Escalation protocols should be employed if Level 3 care is required. A swift, safe transfer to intensive care should take place with close liaison with critical care teams.

Structured review of the critically ill pregnant or postpartum woman

Key components underpinning the ongoing management of women receiving critical care on the labour ward are:

- Use of a dedicated maternity critical care chart (as outlined below)
- Regular structured review

The Structured Review Template (**Figure 2.3**) ensures a structured, comprehensive review of all systems every time the woman is reviewed by the multi-professional team. Such reviews should occur at least 8-hourly.   The template can be provided as a laminated aide memoire on the ward round trolley or provided as a printed sheet for each assessment for filing into the medical records. More detail on the structured review of the critically ill pregnant or postpartum woman is provided in **Section 3**.

Figure 2.3 Maternity Critical Care Structured Review sheet as an 'aide memoire'

Maternal Critical Care Structured review		
This is designed to be used during the multi-professional review of a critically ill pregnant or postpartum woman. ***It does not replace, nor should repeat the observations and information recorded on the Maternal Critical Care chart.*** Relevant notes can be made as each item is considered either directly into the woman's notes or by annotating the work sheet which should be dated, signed and filed in the woman's maternity notes at the end of the review.	**Patient ID (addressograph)** Date........................ Time.....................	

	Items to be considered	Notes:
A	**Airway**	
B	**Breathing** (Respiratory Rate, SpO$_2$, FiO$_2$, chest examination findings)	
C	**Circulation** (Heart rate, BP, capillary refill time, vasopressors)	
D	**Disability** (level of consciousness, pain, epidural or spinal block)	
E	**Electrolytes** (Mg^{2+}, Na$^+$, K$^+$ levels and eGFR/creatinine)	
F	**Fluids** – Review of fluid balance (input, output, blood loss, drains)	
G	**GI & glucose control** (bowel function and gastro-protection measures)	
H	**Haematology** (FBC, clotting profile, VTE prophylaxis)	
I	**Infection** (temperature, Sepsis Six, inflammatory markers, cultures, antibiotics)	
L	**Lines** (cannulae, arterial line, central line, urinary catheter, wound drains)	
M	**Maternal Co-Morbidities** (diabetes, hypertension, asthma, epilepsy)	
N	**Neonatal considerations**	
O	**Obstetric**: antenatal, intrapartum/postpartum related	
P	**Pharmacology** (review drug chart)	
Q	**Questions**	
R	**Recommendations**	
S	**Summary**	
	Signature.. Print.. Date...........................	

Figure 2.4 Maternal Critical Care Chart with guidance for use

The Maternity Critical Care Chart - guidance for use.

RESPIRATORY RATE: This is the single most important parameter for early detection of deterioration and should be documented at all monitoring events.

HEART RATE: Another key sign – tachycardia may be the only sign of deterioration at an early stage. A tachycardic women should be considered hypovolaemic until proven otherwise.

TEMPERATURE: This is not a sensitive marker of deterioration. A temperature rise or fall (>37.5 or <36 °C) may indicate sepsis.

OXYGEN SATURATION: The level of administered oxygen (L/min) or 'air' should be documented with SpO$_2$. Oxygen is prescribed on the drug chart.

BLOOD PRESSURE: Hypotension is a late sign of deterioration as it signifies decompensation and should be taken very seriously. Septic shock can be particularly difficult to recognise, if in doubt perform a venous or arterial blood gas to check pH and lactate. Hypertension is equally important, all pregnant patients with a SBP ≥160mmHg must be treated (MBRRACE – UK 2016).

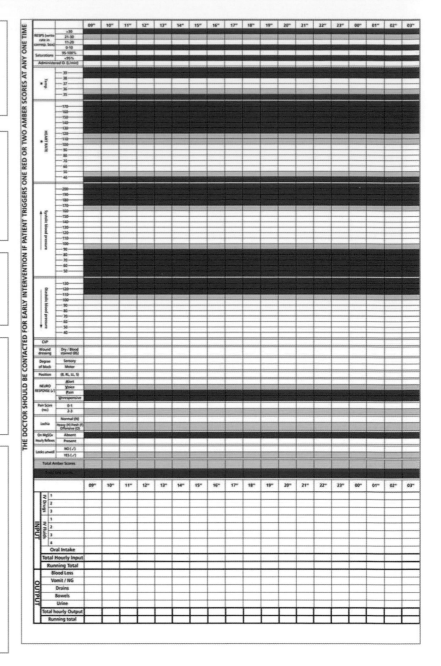

CENTRAL VENOUS PRESSURE: If a patient has a CVP line, ensure the transducer is correctly positioned and zeroed as per the Critical Care Guidelines. Write the CVP reading in the appropriate box.

DEGREE OF BLOCK (in a patient with a spinal or epidural)

MOTOR	SENSORY
1. No foot movement	1. Numb to mid-chest (T4)
2. Slight foot or leg movement	2. Numb to mid-abdomen (T10)
3. Can bend knee or raise leg	3. Numb only below waist (L1)

REFLEXES If a woman is receiving IV magnesium sulfate, the presence or absence of deep tendon reflexes (usually patellar reflex) should be documented hourly.

WOUNDS: Surgical sites should be recorded as dry or bloodstained. Drain losses should be recorded under fluid output.

POSITION Regular changes (minimum 4 hourly) in the woman's position are essential to avoid damage to pressure areas. Right Lateral (RL), Sitting (S), Left Lateral (LL), Back (B)

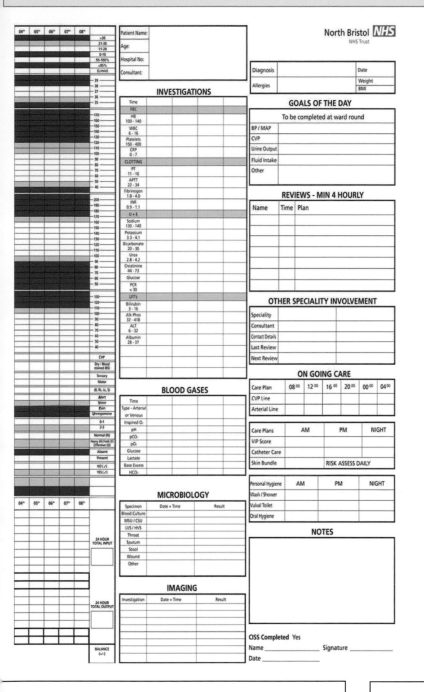

INVESTIGATIONS AND RESULTS: The results of pending investigations (blood tests, imaging and microbiology) should be actively sought and documented on the chart.

NEUROLOGICAL RESPONSE

ALERT: fully awake woman

VOICE: drowsy but answers to name or some kind of response when addressed

PAIN: difficult to rouse, makes a response to sternal rubbing, pinching earlobes or shaking shoulders

UNRESPONSIVE: no response to voice or painful stimulus

AVPU is a measure of the woman's level of consciousness. The best descriptor should be recorded. A fall in AVPU score should always be considered significant. A score of 'P' or below is equivalent to Glasgow coma score of ≤ 8.

All scores should be added up hourly and documented in the same manner as a MOEWS chart. The doctor should be contacted for early intervention IF THE WOMAN TRIGGERS ONE RED OR TWO AMBER AT ANY ONE TIME.

PAIN SCORE Pain scores guide analgesia and adequacy. They should be recorded as 0 (no pain), 1 (mild pain), 2 (moderate pain), 3 (severe pain).

FLUID INPUT This is the volume of all fluid the woman receives including drinking, nasogastric fluids, IV fluids and IV drug infusions. These should be added up to create an hourly total in millilitres (mL), and a running total and recorded on the chart. The 24h total input should be completed at 09.00 every day.

FLUID OUTPUT This is the volume of all fluid the woman loses including urine, blood loss, diarrhoea and vomitus. These should be added up to create an hourly total in millilitres (mL), and a running total and recorded on the chart. The 24h total output should be completed at 09.00 every day.

URINE OUTPUT This is one of the few signs of end organ perfusion. Urine output should be recorded hourly in millilitres (mL) on the chart and contributes to fluid output in the 24h balance.

FLUID BALANCE The fluid balance must be accurate and kept up to date. It is the 24-hour input minus the 24-hour output and should be calculated at 09.00 every day. A new chart is commenced at 09.00 with all fluids starting from zero.

The Maternity Critical Care (MCC) Chart

A Maternity Critical Care Chart (**Figure 2.4**) should be used to document the woman's observations, fluid balance and ongoing clinical investigations, results and medical reviews.

Observations are usually charted hourly, but the frequency at which observations are taken will depend on the clinical condition of the woman. The key observations that should be performed at least hourly are: respiratory rate, oxygen saturation, temperature, heart rate, blood pressure, central venous pressure (if applicable), deep tendon reflexes, fluid input, urine output, fluid output, fluid balance, patient position, neurological response and pain score.

The chart is used to monitor the woman's clinical condition and summarise the results of investigations over a 24-hour period, and a new chart should be commenced at 09:00 each day. An accurately completed maternity critical care chart is key to comprehensively informing regular medical reviews.

Further reading

Knight M, Nair M, Tuffnell D, Kenyon S, Shakespeare J, Brocklehurst P, Kurinczuk JJ (Eds) on behalf of MBRRACE-UK Saving Lives, Improving Mothers' care – Surveillance of maternal deaths in the UK 2012-14 and lessons learned to inform maternity care from the UK and Ireland Confidential Enquiries into Maternal Deaths and morbidity 2009-14. Oxford National Perinatal Epidemiology Unit, University of Oxford 2016: pp 69-75

Knight M, Kenyon S, Brocklehurst P, Neilson J, Shakespeare J, Kurinczuk JJ (Eds.) on behalf of MBRRACE-UK. Saving Lives, Improving Mothers' Care - Lessons learned to inform future maternity care from the UK and Ireland Confidential Enquiries into Maternal Deaths and Morbidity 2009–12. Oxford: National Perinatal Epidemiology Unit, University of Oxford 2014

Royal College of Anaesthetists. Care of the critically ill woman in childbirth; enhanced maternal care 2018. August 2018

Competencies for Recognising and Responding to Acutely Ill Patients in Hospital. *Department of Health,* London 2008
www.dh.gov.uk/en/Publicationsandstatistics/Publications/PublicationsPolicyAndGuidance/DH_096989

Section 3: Structured approach to the review of a critically ill pregnant or postpartum woman

Key Learning Points

- The regular, structured review of the critically ill pregnant or postpartum woman is an essential part of maternal critical care
- A systematic approach should be used to ensure that no key information or interventions are missed
- A complete structured review of critically ill pregnant or postpartum women should be performed at least daily and additionally:
  - Whenever their clinical condition changes
  - When a change in the level of care being provided to the woman is being considered
- High quality critical care often involves providing good basic midwifery, obstetric and anaesthetic care to a consistent standard

It is a common misconception that effective critical care management involves either a highly technological environment (e.g. an intensive care unit), or complicated and invasive interventions. In fact, the critical care interventions with the best evidence base are often those that involve doing the basics consistently and to a high standard. Review of the critically ill pregnant or postpartum woman requires a structured approach to assessment, investigation and management to ensure that no key information or treatments are missed.

This section builds on the structured review introduced in Section 2 (see **Figure 2.3**) and provides more detailed information and guidance on a systematic approach to maternal critical care. By examining each organ system in turn and creating a comprehensive management plan, we can ensure that conditions are optimised for the woman's rapid return to health.

A: Airway

Assessment of the airway is prioritised, as the loss of a pregnant or postpartum woman's airway will rapidly lead to respiratory and then cardiac arrest. The airway can be assessed as follows:

Patent/clear airway:

The vast majority of critically ill pregnant or postpartum women should be able to maintain their own airway without any problem.

Threatened airway:

Snoring, gurgling sounds and the use of neck muscles to aid breathing effort are all signs of a threatened airway. Immediate management involves the application of high-flow oxygen, and summoning urgent help including an anaesthetist. Laying the woman in the recovery position – or flat (with left uterine displacement if antenatal) with simple airway manoeuvres (head tilt and chin lift, or jaw thrust) may successfully relieve the airway obstruction. However, she is likely to require more definitive securing of the airway, which might involve tracheal intubation and transfer to an intensive care unit.

Supported/secured airway:

A supported airway requires an airway manoeuvre (head tilt and chin left, or jaw thrust) to maintain an open airway. A supported airway might also include the use of a nasopharyngeal airway, or an oropharyngeal (Guedel) airway.

A secured airway includes an airway that has been intubated with an endotracheal tube or has a tracheostomy in situ.

Women who have a threatened, supported or secured airway are at significant risk and require the urgent presence of an anaesthetist and consideration for transfer to an intensive care unit.

B: Breathing

Respiratory rate:

A raised respiratory rate is a sensitive marker of organ dysfunction as it often represents an increase in oxygen demand and is therefore an important vital sign to measure. Whilst a raised respiratory rate is sensitive, it is not specific to any particular organ dysfunction (i.e. can occur in respiratory, cardiac, metabolic and other disorders). The normal respiratory rate is 12 to 20. Tachypnoea is defined as a respiratory rate above 20 breaths per minute. Any respiratory rate above 20 requires investigation.

Causes of tachypnoea include:

- pain

- anxiety

- exertion

- respiratory problems: e.g. infection, pulmonary embolus, asthma

- cardiovascular problems: e.g. hypovolaemia, cardiac disease

- metabolic problems: e.g. to compensate for a metabolic acidosis caused by

    o diabetic ketoacidosis in women with diabetes

    o lactic acidosis in sepsis

    o overdose of certain medications

Supplemental oxygen should be considered in all tachypnoeic women.

Respiratory rates above 30 are unusual and require urgent assessment as well as supplemental oxygen. Arterial blood gas (ABG) analysis should also be considered. **Women with respiratory rates above 40 are at risk of tiring due to the effort of maintaining this and an anaesthetic assessment as well as an ABG should be urgently sought.**

A reduced respiratory rate is often due to the effect of medication such as opioids. All routes of opioid administration, including via epidural and spinal, risk causing respiratory depression. A respiratory rate below 8 requires urgent review. Supplemental oxygen should be given, the woman should be stimulated to encourage her to breath, and naloxone (an opioid antagonist) should be considered. Naloxone in this setting is usually given intravenously in the dose of 400mcg, however this dose can also be effective given subcutaneously or IM if there is no intravenous access. It is important to be aware that naloxone has a shorter half-life than most opioids and that vigilance should be maintained for any further respiratory depression; if this occurs a repeat dose of naloxone can be administered.

Oxygen saturations:

Modern pulse oximeters can give an accurate measurement of how saturated the woman's blood is with oxygen. However, they are less accurate in certain conditions, for example: if the probe is not attached properly, the woman is shivering or fitting, the woman has very cold/shut-down peripheries or the probe's light signal cannot pass through the finger easily because of coloured nail varnish or dressings.

All pulse oximeter readings should be considered in the context of how much oxygen the woman is receiving. Normal saturations (> 97%) are only normal if they are maintained while the woman is breathing room air. Therefore, the amount of oxygen they are receiving (FiO_2) should also be documented and taken into account – for example, it is extremely concerning if a woman's oxygen saturations are only 94% on 50% O_2. Any woman with abnormally low oxygen saturations should be urgently reviewed by an anaesthetist.

Oxygen saturations should not be relied upon alone to assess the adequacy of ventilation. It is possible to have significant respiratory depression and maintain normal oxygen saturations, particularly if the woman is receiving supplemental oxygen. Therefore, respiratory rate is usually a more sensitive marker.

Fraction of inspired oxygen (FiO_2):

The FiO_2 describes the inspired oxygen concentration and is classically given as a fraction of 1.0 (FiO_2 of 1.0 = 100% oxygen) but is often signified as a percentage (e.g. room air has an FiO_2 of 0.21, which is 21% oxygen). As it is difficult to accurately measure the FiO_2 without specialist equipment, on a labour ward, the flow rate of oxygen (L/min) is often measured and documented instead.

As a rough guide:

- 2 L/min of oxygen gives approximately 28% O_2 (FiO_2 = 0.28)
- 5 L/min is approximately 40% O_2 (FiO_2 = 0.4)
- 10 L/min is approximately 60% O_2 (FiO_2 = 0.6)

A non-rebreather facemask has a reservoir of oxygen, and if correctly applied with a flow of 10–15 L/min of oxygen, it can give approximately 80–90% O_2 (FiO_2 0.8–0.9). More information on modes of oxygen delivery is provided in Section 4.

High inspired levels of oxygen should only be used for a short period of time, e.g. during the initial resuscitation of a sick pregnant or postpartum woman. Thereafter, the flows should be reduced to maintain the oxygen saturations recommended by the team managing the woman. If high oxygen levels (e.g. 5 L/min O_2, equivalent to 40% O_2) are needed to achieve this, the woman should be reviewed as she may need further optimisation of their respiratory function. This might include medical therapy, humidified oxygen, non-invasive ventilation or even invasive ventilation (via an endotracheal tube) and may require transfer to intensive care.

Examination findings:

The woman's respiratory effort should be noted, including whether they need to adopt more efficient postures to breath (e.g. sitting forward with arms resting on legs) and whether they need to use accessory muscles (e.g. neck muscles). Engaging the woman in conversation can help determine whether she can complete sentences without taking an extra breath. The presence of any central cyanosis (i.e. blue-ish coloured lips) should be recognised. Asthmatic women should have their peak expiratory flow rate (PEFR) regularly checked and documented.

Shortness of breath may also be a symptom of cardiovascular disease; MBRRACE-UK highlighted that any woman with persistent shortness of breath when lying flat warrants urgent review to investigate potential cardiac disease (1).

The chest should be auscultated during medical reviews. The chest should be examined for expansion and auscultation in the sitting position (if possible), including checking both lung bases and axillae. Percussion note and vocal resonance should also be considered, based on other examination findings.

C: Cardiovascular system

Heart rate:

Heart rate is another non-specific marker of organ dysfunction; like respiratory rate it increases as oxygen demand increases, however it is less sensitive, needing larger physiological derangements before the woman becomes tachycardic. Heart rate can also be increased by pain and anxiety.

Tachycardia is defined as a heart rate ≥ 100 beats per minute. A maternal tachycardia is most commonly associated with hypovolaemia from haemorrhage and a potential source of bleeding must therefore be investigated alongside initiation of treatment. However, the heart rate will also increase in response to increased oxygen demand from respiratory, cardiac, metabolic and other causes. Whilst it may be worth considering whether the tachycardia is a side effect of any medication that has been administered e.g. salbutamol or magnesium sulfate, other medical causes must be ruled out before accepting this as an explanation.

A persistent tachycardia of over 120 bpm is unusual and should prompt an urgent medical review. Intravenous access should be obtained and consideration given to administering a bolus of intravenous fluids (e.g. 250–500 mL of a balanced crystalloid such as Hartmann's solution). Bloods should be taken to check haemoglobin, U&Es, inflammatory markers, coagulation, lactate and a group and screen. Supplemental oxygen may be helpful.

A tachycardia of over 150 bpm may be due to an abnormal heart rhythm, or severe organ dysfunction. High-flow oxygen should be given whilst urgent help is obtained. IV access should be established, and bloods sent as above. Arterial or venous blood gas levels may be useful. A 3-lead

ECG may give an indication of the cause of the heart rhythm, but a 12-lead ECG will often give more information. More information on ECG monitoring is provided in Section 5.

Bradycardia is defined as a heart rate less than 60, however this can be normal in many fit, young women. A heart rate less than 40 is unusual and usually warrants urgent clinical review. Significant bradycardia may be caused by a vagal reflex (e.g. during a faint or from cervical shock), by medication, spinal or epidural analgesia, electrolyte imbalance, or occasionally by an abnormal heart rhythm such as heart block.

Any woman with an abnormal heart rate should also have their blood pressure checked. Hypotension in the context of tachycardia or bradycardia is an ominous sign and needs urgent multi-professional review.

Blood pressure:

The systolic blood pressure (SBP) is the maximal pressure generated in the arteries with each heartbeat. The diastolic blood pressure (DBP) is the pressure in the arteries during diastole when the heart is relaxed. The mean arterial pressure (MAP) is the average pressure within the arteries during the cardiac cycle and is equivalent to the end-organ pressure. Whilst the diastolic blood pressure in women with pre-eclampsia has been traditionally used to monitor progress of the disease and its fetal effects, systolic blood pressure is now widely recognised as more important in terms of both maternal hypertension and hypotension. Both the systolic and diastolic blood pressure readings must always be documented and communicated.

Hypotension can be variably defined, but a systolic blood pressure below 100 mmHg is unusual and warrants a more detailed review. A systolic blood pressure below 90 mmHg should not be ignored and should prompt a multi-professional review. Blood pressure is affected by pregnancy and it is always useful to check the woman's booking and most recent blood pressure readings from her antenatal notes.

Hypotension due to hypovolaemia from haemorrhage is a late sign and may signify blood loss in excess of 30% of the circulating blood volume, even if the source of the bleeding is not immediately apparent. Hypotension can also occur in the context of sepsis. If a septic woman remains hypotensive after a 'fluid challenge' then they are likely to be suffering from 'septic shock'. This has a high mortality rate and needs urgent referral to the critical care team whilst multi-professional management according to the Sepsis Six and the Surviving Sepsis Care Bundle (see Section 9) is ongoing.

Severe systolic hypertension with systolic BP > 150 mmHg should be avoided. In the context of pre-eclampsia a systolic BP of ≥ 160 mmHg is associated with an increased risk of intracerebral haemorrhage; the risks are increased in pre-eclampsia due to endothelial dysfunction that predisposes to vascular permeability (leaky vessels). Severe systolic hypertension in pre-eclampsia should be treated promptly. The management of pre-eclampsia and Eclampsia, including severe hypertension is covered in Module 6 of the PROMPT Course Manual (Third Edition).

When documenting the maternal blood pressure, it is important to note if any medication that could alter the blood pressure e.g. vasopressors, inotropes or anti-hypertensives have been administered.

Vasopressors:

These are medications that act to increase the blood pressure through vasoconstriction. Those most commonly used in pregnant and postpartum women tend to be α-agonists such as phenylephrine and metaraminol; these may cause a reflex bradycardia when given. Mixed α- and β-agonists such as ephedrine may also be used; these have a tendency to cause a tachycardia through their β-agonist effects. More potent vasoconstrictors such as noradrenaline (norepinephrine) are rarely used in pregnancy and postpartum and require administration through a central line. When any vasopressor infusion is administered it requires frequent (e.g. initially every 5 minutes) blood pressure monitoring.

Inotropes:

These are medications that are given to increase the force of contraction of the heart and are often β-agonists such as dobutamine and adrenaline. They are potent medicines that require intensive monitoring and are rarely used outside of intensive care and coronary care units.

Capillary refill time:

This is a way of assessing peripheral blood flow and is prolonged in states of hypovolaemia (e.g. haemorrhage, or functional hypovolaemia due to central vasodilatation in sepsis), dehydration and hypothermia. The capillary refill time is best assessed centrally (e.g. by pressing on the sternum for 5 seconds and counting the time for the skin to return to the same colour as the surrounding area) as this is less affected by cold than the fingers. A normal capillary refill time is less than 2 seconds.

Central venous pressure (CVP):

If a CVP line is present, the CVP should be checked during each clinical review. Ensure the transducer is level with the right atrium of the heart. Trends in CVP are often more useful than absolute numbers. A rising CVP suggests that the right side of the heart is becoming fuller, either due to an increased venous fluid volume, or due to the heart being unable to empty effectively (e.g. in heart failure). A falling CVP suggests hypovolaemia and represents ongoing haemorrhage until proven otherwise. A CVP line can be particularly useful to guide fluid replacement in cases of haemorrhage where the woman also has impaired kidney function, e.g. due to pre-eclampsia, as there is a risk of causing pulmonary oedema.

Examination findings:

- It is useful to check the woman's peripheries (fingers and toes) to feel if they are cold (as occurs in hypovolaemia, hypothermia, or peripheral vasoconstriction) or warm and well perfused.
- Skin colour and the presence of mottling can also give information about the adequacy of peripheral circulation.
- Looking at the woman's tongue and mucous membranes (lips and lining of the cheeks) can help identify dehydration.
- Dependent areas (feet if sitting or standing, sacral area if in bed) should be checked for oedema.
- Examining the woman's conjunctivae may help to identify anaemia.
- Heart sounds should be auscultated.
- The jugular venous pressure should be assessed to help establish the woman's volume status.

A recent MBRRACE-UK report also identified that any woman who is noted to have persistent shortness of breath when lying flat should also warrant urgent review, as this may be a symptom of cardiac disease (1).

D: Disability

The brain's function is normally maintained even when unwell, so any change in consciousness level is a red flag (1) and warrants urgent senior multi-professional review. The assessment of a fall in consciousness level should aim to identify and treat the underlying cause (e.g. hypovolaemia, sepsis); if thought to be from a neurological cause this would usually require urgent brain imaging with a CT scan or MRI.

AVPU:

A – Alert

V – responds to Voice

P – responds to Pain

U – Unconscious

This is a useful quick assessment of global consciousness level. Women who score 'P' or less are profoundly obtunded (equivalent to a GCS of 8/15) and are likely to need intubation to protect their airway.

Glasgow Coma Score (GCS):

This 15-point scale gives a more detailed and objective assessment of consciousness level (see Section 8). A GCS of 15/15 is expected in virtually all women; a fall in GCS by even one point requires urgent review. A woman with a GCS of ≤ 8/15 may be unable to maintain her own airway, and hence will probably need intubation. A GCS of 3/15 is the lowest score possible and represents profound unconsciousness.

Pupil size and reaction:

Pupils should be equal in size and in their reaction to light. A single dilated pupil, in the presence of a fall in consciousness level is due to raised intracranial pressure (e.g. from an intracerebral bleed) until proven otherwise. Bilaterally dilated pupils are often caused by catecholamines (e.g. pain, anxiety, medication) whilst bilaterally constricted pupils can be seen as a result of opioid use/overdose.

Pain:

Pain scores should be assessed and appropriate analgesics prescribed and given. Pain scores that are persistently higher than expected should trigger an obstetric review to rule out any treatable cause for the pain, e.g. an expanding haematoma.

Epidural/spinal block level:

Both the sensory and motor degree of the block should be assessed. Once a block is established, the sensory level should be symmetrical and relatively stable. The motor block from an epidural may become more dense as the amount of administered local anaesthetic accumulates. Once the block has been discontinued, the sensory and motor function should gradually return to normal.

If the block does not recede as expected, request an anaesthetic review. A persistent or evolving significant motor block, especially if unilateral, may be due to a haematoma or abscess in the vertebral canal. Rapid assessment and management is vital, as permanent neurological injury can occur if this is not surgically decompressed within hours. Therefore, an immediate anaesthetic review is required as the woman may need urgent MRI imaging and transfer to a neurosurgical centre.

High spinal block and local anaesthetic toxicity are anaesthetic emergencies that require a coordinated multi-professional approach. The management of these emergencies are detailed in Module 4 of the PROMPT Course Manual (Third Edition).

Tendon reflexes:

Women receiving a magnesium sulfate infusion should have their deep tendon reflexes checked regularly. Magnesium excess is rarely a problem in women with normal kidney function, but signs of magnesium toxicity include visual disturbances, flushing, muscle weakness and respiratory depression. Intravenous calcium (10 mL 10% calcium gluconate (or 5-10 mL 10% calcium chloride if this is unavailable) slow IV) should be available to treat magnesium toxicity.

E: Electrolytes

Critically ill women should have their urea and electrolytes (U&Es) checked daily to assess their renal function. Other electrolytes such as magnesium may also need to be checked. Any woman with impaired renal function should have their medication chart reviewed for potentially nephrotoxic drugs, e.g. non-steroidal anti-inflammatory drugs (NSAIDs), and aminoglycoside antibiotics such as gentamicin. Also, renally-excreted drugs, e.g. low-molecular weight heparins (LMWHs) such as enoxaparin (Clexane®) and tinzaparin may need their doses adjusted.

Urea:

Urea is a waste product from the metabolism of nitrogen-containing compounds in the body. It is excreted by the kidneys in the urine and therefore may accumulate in renal failure. A rising urea with a normal creatinine may be an indication of dehydration. An isolated raised urea can also occur due to an excess of nitrogen absorption from the bowel, as occurs in upper gastro-intestinal haemorrhage (digested red blood cells are a rich source of nitrogen).

Creatinine:

Creatinine is produced from skeletal muscle breakdown and is also excreted by the kidneys. A rise in creatinine is most often seen in renal impairment as the kidneys are unable to excrete it effectively. An outline of acute kidney injury (AKI) is given in **Box 3.1**. Rarely, a raised creatinine can be due to excessive skeletal muscle breakdown, as can occur secondary to immobility, muscle injury, or deep-seated infection (e.g. necrotising fasciitis).

'Pre-renal' renal failure

- Inadequate perfusion of the kidneys
  - e.g. hypovolaemia, severe dehydration
- Treatment involves optimising circulating volume and renal perfusion by judicious boluses of intravenous fluids

'Renal' renal failure

- Damage to, or disease of, kidney tissue or vasculature
  - e.g. acute tubular necrosis, pre-eclampsia, medication (e.g. NSAIDs), infection (e.g. pyelonephritis)
  - Treatment depends upon the cause

'Post-renal' renal failure

- Obstruction of the urinary tract, leading to back-pressure of urine on the kidneys:
  - e.g. blocked catheter, ureteric injury, renal or ureteric stones
- Treatment is by relieving the obstruction, e.g. by replacing the urinary catheter, inserting a ureteric stent

Sodium:

Sodium is the main extracellular cation (positively charged ion) and its levels are usually tightly maintained. A low sodium (hyponatraemia is $Na^+ < 135$ mmol/L, severe hyponatraemia is $Na^+ < 120$ mmol/L) may be caused by a rapid and excessive sodium loss, e.g. *early* effect of vomiting, diarrhoea, diuretics. Hyponatraemia can also be caused by adrenal insufficiency or dilution from excessive water intake (oral intake, or intravenous free water, e.g. from 5% dextrose/glucose solution); in these situations, the urine will also be dilute. In the syndrome of inappropriate ADH secretion (SIADH), the sodium in the blood is diluted by excessive water retention driven by the kidneys; in this situation the urine will be concentrated. The management of hyponatraemia is complex and requires treatment of the underlying cause, alongside very gradual correction of fluid balance and sodium levels.

Hypernatraemia ($Na^+ > 145$ mmol/L, severe hypernatraemia $Na^+ > 160$ mmol/L) most frequently occurs due to loss of water (dehydration), especially with *continued* vomiting, diarrhoea and diuretics. Hypernatremia can also occur due to excessive sodium administration from inappropriate IV fluids (e.g. 0.9% NaCl) or excessive sodium retention (e.g. hyperaldosteronism). Diabetes insipidus is caused by too little or ineffective anti-diuretic hormone (ADH), meaning that water is not appropriately retained from the kidneys and can lead to hypernatraemia with very dilute urine. Its management involves the gradual restoration of circulating volume and sodium levels, with treatment of the underlying cause.

Potassium:

Potassium is the main intracellular cation, and its levels are also tightly maintained in health. Hypokalaemia ($K^+ < 3.5$ mmol/L, severe hypokalaemia is $K^+ \leq 2.5$ mmol/L) can be caused by potassium loss from diarrhoea, diuretics or steroid use. Changes in plasma potassium concentration can have profound effects on cardiac rhythm. Hypokalaemia can cause bradycardia, ST segment depression and inverted T-waves on the ECG; and if left untreated can lead to asystole. Intravenous access and cardiac monitoring are important. The potassium should be gradually raised by oral or intravenous potassium (NB – intravenous potassium can lead to cardiac arrest if given rapidly; infusions are usually limited to 10 mmol/hour).

Hyperkalaemia ($K^+ > 5.0$ mmol/L, moderate hyperkalaemia is K^+ 6.0–6.4 mmol/L, severe hyperkalaemia is $K^+ \geq 6.5$ mmol/L) can occur with renal impairment, skeletal muscle breakdown, and drugs such as spironolactone. A common cause of raised K^+ in a blood sample is the cellular breakdown of red blood cells during the taking of the blood test: if unsure, send an urgent arterial or venous blood sample to confirm whether the hyperkalaemia is true before excluding it.

The main risk with hyperkalaemia is life-threatening cardiac rhythm abnormalities. The first sign on the ECG is tall, tented T-waves; if the hyperkalaemia is untreated, QRS and ST changes may occur, before progressing to cardiac arrest from ventricular fibrillation or asystole.

The emergency management of hyperkalaemia involves protecting the heart from the effects of the high potassium levels (e.g. by giving 10 mL of 10% calcium gluconate (or 5 - 10 mL 10% calcium chloride)), giving medication that drives potassium into the cells (e.g. salbutamol or insulin), and promoting the reduction of the plasma potassium load (e.g. by chelating agents, such as calcium resonium; or by dialysis): see **Box 3.2**.

- Perform 12-lead ECG and attach 3-lead ECG monitoring

- If potassium > 6.5 mmol/L, ECG changes, or symptomatic:

    1. **Protect the heart**: 10mL of 10% calcium gluconate/chloride slow IV injection, repeat at 5-minute intervals until ECG has normalised

    2. **Shift potassium into cells:**

        - **(a)**: nebulised salbutamol 5 –10 mg

        - **(b)**: 10 units soluble insulin (e.g. human actrapid) in 50mL 50% dextrose/glucose administered via a large vein over 20 minutes

    3. **Stop potassium containing/retaining drugs**: review drug chart and stop any medications containing or retaining potassium

    4. **Remove potassium from the body**: promote diuresis with fluids, consider diuretics and calcium resonium. Consider renal replacement therapy (e.g. haemofiltration or haemodialysis) if hyperkalaemia is resistant to above measures – discuss with renal physician and/or intensive care specialist

Estimated Glomerular Filtration Rate (eGFR):

eGFR is a calculated number which gives an indication of overall renal function and is based on the serum creatinine and a number of other variables. A reduction in eGFR is associated with worsening kidney function; in the non-pregnant population it can be used to stratify the severity of kidney disease and may be used to make recommendations about reducing drug dosages if the kidney disease is severe enough. However, owing to the physiological changes of pregnancy, eGFR is not recommended for use with pregnant or postpartum women as the test will over- or under-estimate the eGFR depending on which calculation your laboratory uses to derive it. So, whilst eGFR in maternal critical care may show useful trends, its values should be interpreted with caution.

Magnesium:

Magnesium is a predominantly, intracellular cation (positive ion), which is involved in many physiological processes. Its main actions are exerted by opposing calcium-sensing receptors within cells, and so it can be considered an intracellular calcium antagonist. Overall its actions tend towards membrane stabilisation (hence its use in eclampsia prophylaxis and treatment, cerebral neuroprotection in preterm infants and use as an anti-arrhythmic and analgesic agent), or smooth muscle relaxation (e.g. uterine relaxation, reducing blood pressure, bronchodilation).

When given therapeutically, levels of magnesium tend to lead to serum magnesium levels above the normal range of 0.8–1.0 mmol/L. For example, for seizure prophylaxis in severe pre-eclampsia, suggested therapeutic levels are in the range of 2–4 mmol/L. However, magnesium toxicity can occur in women with renal impairment (as may occur in severe pre-eclampsia) and so the monitoring of deep tendon reflexes and urine output is vital. Progressively high levels of magnesium lead to increasing muscle weakness, respiratory embarrassment and loss of consciousness. The emergency management of magnesium toxicity involves giving intravenous calcium: 10 mL of 10% calcium gluconate (or 5 – 10 mL 10% calcium chloride) by slow IV injection.

Hypomagnesaemia (Mg^{2+} < 0.7 mmol/L) is frequently seen alongside hypokalaemia and may be caused by low magnesium intake or absorption; or losses from diarrhoea, renal impairment and drugs such as diuretics. The management is by oral or intravenous replacement.

F: Fluids

Critically ill pregnant or postpartum women should have regular recording of all fluid inputs and outputs on an hourly basis, and the difference between these (the fluid balance).

Fluid intake:

Fluid intakes include oral fluids, enteral nutrition, intravenous fluids and fluids given with medication. Intravenous fluids include crystalloids, colloids and blood products. Crystalloids are fluids containing dissolved salts or sugars in water and can be further categorised into isotonic crystalloids (e.g. Hartmann's solution and 0.9% NaCl) and hypotonic crystalloids (e.g. 5% Dextrose). Isotonic crystalloids are the mainstay of intravenous fluid supplementation and are used for both fluid resuscitation and maintenance of fluid administration in a pregnant or post-partum woman who is unable to take adequate fluid orally. Balanced crystalloids such as Hartmann's or Plasma-lyte are preferable to 0.9% Sodium Chloride (NaCl) as they avoid the hyperchloraemic metabolic acidosis associated with 0.9% NaCl.

Colloids are fluids with small particles held in suspension; they include human albumin solution (HAS) and semi-synthetic solutions (e.g. gelatins and starches). The semi-synthetic colloids are associated with adverse outcomes when used in critical illness, especially sepsis, and therefore, should generally be avoided. Human albumin solution may have a role in large volume fluid resuscitation in sepsis that may be typical of a pregnant or post-partum woman who needs aggressive critical care management.

Fluid output:

Fluid output includes all fluid loses. Critically ill pregnant or postpartum women should have a urinary catheter in situ to accurately measure their hourly urine output; an acceptable hourly urine output is > 0.5 mL/kg/hr (this will differ in women with pre-eclampsia where a more conservative urine output will be acceptable). Other fluid loses include those from drains, vomiting, NG tubes and diarrhoea – these should all be charted on a regular basis.

Fluid balance:

The difference between fluid intake and output is the fluid balance, this should be charted as a running total and then reset every 24 hours (e.g. at 09:00). This allows an assessment of the overall fluid losses and gains the pregnant or post-partum woman is making. In health, fluid losses and intake should be approximately equal, and the body maintains a neutral fluid balance. During critical illness it is important to monitor (and potentially manipulate) the body's fluid balance; an excessively negative fluid balance can lead to dehydration, hypovolaemia and renal injury. A positive fluid balance may be required during the resuscitation phase of many acute illnesses but can then lead to oedema, and the other adverse effects of excess body fluid on multiple organ systems. Women with pre-eclampsia are very sensitive to excess body fluid and therefore close monitoring of their fluid balance is vital.

Bear in mind that a fluid balance chart doesn't consider insensible (unmeasurable) fluid losses such as from faeces, sweat and respiration; these are approximately 300–500 mL/day in health, but may be more in critical illness. Therefore, a careful *clinical* assessment of the woman and their volume status is vital.

G: GI & Glucose control

The gastrointestinal tract should be fully assessed for function and to minimise complications of critical illness. This should start with an assessment of symptoms including nausea, vomiting, abdominal pain and bowel opening (frequency and nature) and a physical examination assessing for any signs of intra-abdominal pathology and the nature of any surgical wounds and drains. The nutritional state of the woman should be monitored, and it should be noted how nutrition is being delivered. In women who are not expected to achieve adequate nutritional intake within three days, supplemental enteral nutrition should be considered.

Ileus (absence of gastrointestinal motility) is common during critical illness and may present with vomiting and large gastric aspirates if an NG tube is in place. It is important to maintain the overall fluid balance if these losses are large. The continued use of gentle enteral feed helps forward motion and motility simulants can be considered (e.g. metoclopramide). Diarrhoea is commonly caused by infection or as a side-effect of drugs e.g. antibiotics or laxatives. Stool samples should be sent to the laboratory for M, C & S and for *C. difficile* toxin. Failure to open bowels is common and is usually related to ileus, drugs such opiates and lack of enteral nutrition. It is important to clinically exclude bowel obstruction, ensure adequate hydration and commence laxatives. Liver function tests should be monitored as any abnormal results may indicate HELLP syndrome.

Gastric protection:

Critically ill pregnant and postpartum women are potentially at risk of stress ulcer formation and subsequent gastrointestinal haemorrhage; additional risk factors include underlying coagulopathy, mechanical ventilation and failure to achieve enteral nutrition. These women should receive stress ulcer prophylaxis in the form of either a proton pump inhibitor or a H_2-receptor antagonist.

Glucose control:

Critical illness leads to a stress response and this in turn can induce hyperglycaemia, including in non-diabetic women. High blood glucose is associated with poorer outcomes during critical illness and therefore blood sugars should be controlled. There is also evidence that targeting very tight glycaemic control can be harmful through increased episodes of hypoglycaemia. Critically ill pregnant and postpartum women should have their glucose maintained between 6–10 mmol/L (although 4–12 mmol/L is acceptable); this is usually achieved using a variable rate insulin infusion and should be considered when the blood glucose is consistently > 10 mmol/L.

H: Haematology

On a daily basis the haematological profile of the critically ill woman should be monitored with a full blood count (FBC) and a clotting profile.

A low haemoglobin concentration is a measure of anaemia and there are multiple causes in the pregnant or postpartum woman. Mild anaemia may be physiological due to the dilutional effects of pregnancy. More significant anaemia may be as a result of haemorrhage, haemolysis (for example HELLP syndrome) or the effects of bone marrow suppression during critical illness. In the stable critically ill woman a transfusion threshold of 70 g/L is acceptable. In women with active haemorrhage, blood products need to be administered depending on the rate of haemorrhage and the physiological state of the woman.

Platelet Disorders:

Thrombocytopenia is rarely symptomatic until the platelet count is < 50×10^9/L. There are multiple causes in the pregnant or postpartum woman including pregnancy related conditions (HELLP

46

syndrome, pre-eclampsia and pregnancy induced thrombocytopenia), haemorrhage, disseminated intravascular coagulation (DIC) and sepsis. Management includes treating any underlying precipitant. For women who are not bleeding and are critically ill, the platelet count should be maintained above 20 x 10^9/L. Women with thrombocytopenia should be discussed with the haemotologist to add their management. Obstetric and anaesthetic involvement is important; especially if birth, surgery or regional anaesthesia (spinal or epidural) are planned.

Coagulation Disorders:

Coagulopathy in the critically ill pregnant or postpartum woman can be caused by multiple conditions including HELLP syndrome, severe pre-eclampsia, haemorrhage, DIC, severe sepsis and liver failure. The management of coagulopathy will depend on whether there is bleeding or not and may require the transfusion of various blood products (e.g. fresh frozen plasma and cryoprecipitate/fibrinogen concentrate) depending on the results of coagulation tests (including fibrinogen).

All critically ill pregnant and postpartum women are at increased risk of venous thromboembolic disease (VTE); they should undergo a risk assessment and receive appropriate prophylaxis including mechanical (compression stockings and sequential mechanical compression devices) and pharmacological (e.g. low molecular weight heparin) measures if there are no contraindications.

I: Infection

The daily assessment of the critically ill pregnant or postpartum woman should include an assessment for any new infections and the management of known infections. This includes review of the woman's temperature (looking for fever > 38 °C or hypothermia < 36 °C); clinical assessment looking for signs or symptoms of infection, for example, in the respiratory tract, genitourinary tract, surgical site wounds and invasive lines and finally a review of laboratory data including daily inflammatory markers – white cell count (WCC) and C-reactive protein (CRP). Results of any recent microbiological samples should also be reviewed along with current antimicrobial therapy including the duration of that therapy and intended stop date.

If there is evidence of new infection or untreated infection, for example fever, abnormal inflammatory markers and new or deteriorating clinical symptoms and signs, then the source of infection should be investigated (e.g. radiological imaging, microbiological samples – blood, sputum, urine cultures and swabs if indicated) and the antimicrobial therapy reviewed in consultation with local guidelines and microbiologists. It is important in all cases of infection to achieve source control and to promptly initiate antibiotic therapy if sepsis is suspected in line with the Surviving Sepsis Guidelines (see Section 9).

L: Lines

Each day the critically ill pregnant or postpartum woman should have an assessment of any indwelling devices including peripheral and central venous cannulae, arterial cannulae, drains, urinary catheters and epidural catheters. This assessment should look for complications e.g. infection, pain or malfunction and assessment of the need for each indwelling device and consideration of its suitability for removal.

M: Maternal medicine

A thorough history should be sought for any critically ill pregnant or postpartum woman and significant past medical history highlighted. It is important to ensure that any co-morbid diseases are managed in conjunction with the critical illness. An assessment of any medical co-morbidities should be made, including the impact on the current critical illness and a review of any pre-existing treatments. It is often possible (and advisable) to continue long-term treatments but depending on the complexity of the co-morbid disease it may be necessary to seek advice from relevant clinical specialists and the pharmacist.

N: Neonatal/fetal considerations

If the critically ill woman is pregnant, careful thought should be given to the fetal condition during every review. Decisions should be made and reconsidered as to how the fetal condition should be monitored (e.g. electronic fetal monitoring, liquor volume and umbilical artery dopplers) and how often these should take place. Plans should be made in advance as to what action should occur if there is an acute deterioration in the fetal condition. Would it be safe to perform a Category 1 caesarean section for suspected fetal compromise, or would that be too risky for the mother? Logistically, monitoring the fetal condition and expediting an emergency birth can be more complex if the woman is being cared for in ICU, as this may be situated some distance from the regular obstetric and neonatal facilities.

If a woman is deteriorating, the birth of the baby is likely to improve the maternal condition. A discussion should take place between the obstetricians, anaesthetists, neonatologists, and other relevant specialities, together with the parents, regarding the need to expedite birth. However, the maternal condition should always take precedence over the risks to the baby.

If the woman is postpartum, then it is useful to know the condition of the newborn baby, for example, is the baby being treated for sepsis and are there any positive neonatal cultures? It is likely that both mother and baby will have the same organisms. Similarly, the neonatal team should be informed of any positive cultures from the mother, as the neonate may need to start or change antibiotic treatment.

O: Obstetric

Obstetric issues should be considered at every review. For example:

- Are corticosteroids required to aid fetal lung maturity? Are there any contraindications?
- Should magnesium sulfate be given for neuroprotection of the fetus?
- How often is fetal monitoring being undertaken and what is the plan if there are concerns over the fetal condition?
- Should medical thromboprophylaxis be continued, and in what form, and at what time?
- Is the postpartum uterus well contracted?

P: Pharmacology

Each day as part of the ward round, the woman's medication chart should be reviewed. The purpose of this review is to discover any prescription or dosing errors, any medications that have not been given and the reason why, and also any medications that need reviewing and potentially discontinuing or modifying. A review of any admission medications is vital too, to reconcile the medication chart where possible.

Summary and Recommendations

At the end of the systematic review of the pregnant or postpartum woman the key problems for that day should be summarised.

A treatment plan for that day should then be documented and clearly communicated with the clinical team and the pregnant or postpartum woman.

At least one 'Goal of the Day' should be set so that all staff are aware of how the care of the woman should be moving forward. Example 'Goals of the Day' might be:

1. Aim to keep systolic blood pressure between 130–150mmHg
2. Aim for a urine output greater than 100 mL over four hours
3. Sit out in a chair for at least one hour
4. Visit baby in the neonatal unit

Reference

1. Knight M, Nair M, Tuffnell D, Kenyon S, Shakespeare J, Brocklehurst P, Kurinczuk JJ (Eds) on behalf of MBRRACE-UK Saving Lives, Improving Mothers' care – Surveillance of maternal deaths in the UK 2012-14 and lessons learned to inform maternity care from the UK and Ireland Confidential Enquiries into Maternal Deaths and morbidity 2009-14. Oxford National Perinatal Epidemiology Unit, University of Oxford 2016: pp 1 - 120

Section 4: Oxygen administration and blood gas interpretation

> **Key Learning Points**
>
> - Supplemental oxygen can be useful in the management of many critically ill pregnant or postpartum women
> - Oxygen is a medication, and should be prescribed
> - The amount of oxygen delivered depends on the flow-rate, and the type of device being used
> - Arterial blood gases give information both on respiratory function, and how well the body's tissues are coping with critical illness
> - Type I respiratory failure occurs with inadequate oxygenation
> - Type II respiratory failure and respiratory acidosis occur with inadequate ventilation
> - Metabolic acidosis is usually caused by inadequate tissue perfusion

Oxygen is required for the functioning and survival of all body tissues. Oxygen should be regarded as a medication and should be prescribed accordingly. Prescriptions should include:

- Flow rate
- Delivery system
- Duration of therapy
- Instructions for monitoring.

> **In an emergency situation (e.g. cardiac or respiratory arrest, acute hypoxia) oxygen should be administered immediately without waiting for a prescription**

When should oxygen be used?

- Hypoxia* or hypoxaemia[§]
  - Oxygen saturations < 94% (or possibly < 91% if the woman has pre-existing respiratory disease)

o The partial pressure of oxygen (PaO$_2$ – a measure of dissolved oxygen in arterial blood) is less than 10 kPa on an arterial blood gas (ABG)

- Acute hypotension
- Breathing inadequacy
- Sepsis
- Acute illness
- Severe anaemia
- During the peri-operative period

* 'Hypoxia' means there is insufficient oxygen reaching the body's cells to maintain their normal function. Hypoxia may be signified by a raised serum lactate.

§ 'Hypoxaemia' is low levels of oxygen in the blood (PaO$_2$ < 10 kPa).

Signs and symptoms of hypoxia

- Low oxygen saturations
- Increased respiratory rate and heart rate
- Restlessness and changes in level of consciousness
- Cyanosis (blue lips and nail beds)
- Chest pain

Oxygen delivery devices

Non-rebreather facemask (with reservoir bag)

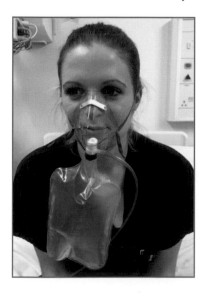

- Delivers high concentrations of oxygen (85% at 15 L/min)
- Has a bag which acts as a reservoir of oxygen
- One-way valves on the mask prevent room air from diluting the oxygen concentration given to the woman
- A tight seal is essential
- ***The reservoir bag must be expanded before use***. The reservoir bag should be sufficiently inflated by turning the oxygen on and covering the one-way valve inside the mask with your thumb until the bag is about two-thirds full. The mask can then be fitted to the woman.

Simple (Hudson) facemask

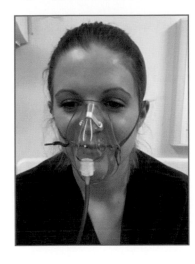

- Easy to use
- Requires a good fit
- The volume of the facemask is 100–300 mL
- It delivers 40–60% oxygen when using flowrates of 5 to 10 L/min
- The concentration of oxygen delivered is influenced by respiratory rate, tidal volume and underlying pathology
- However, the facemask can be obtrusive, uncomfortable and confining. It muffles communication, obstructs coughing and impedes eating

Nasal cannulae

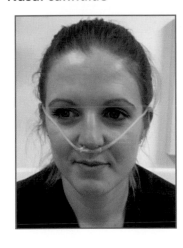

- Easy to use and generally well tolerated
- Comfortable for long periods
- Woman can eat and talk easily
- Possible to deliver oxygen concentrations of 24–40% when using flowrates of 1–6 L/min
- Flow rates in excess of 4 L/min may cause discomfort and drying of mucous membranes

Venturi mask

- Mixes a specific volume of air and oxygen and is useful for accurately delivering fixed concentrations of oxygen.
- Valves are colour-coded and the oxygen flow rate required to deliver a specific concentration is shown on each valve.
- Can deliver titratable oxygen concentrations between 24–60%.
- Important to recognise that the percentage of oxygen delivered by the valve should be recorded, not the flow rate, as looking at the flow rate alone does not reflect the amount of oxygen being delivered to the woman

Humidification circuit
- Is recommended if more than 4 L/min of oxygen is being delivered for a prolonged period.
- Helps prevent drying of mucous membranes.
- Helps encourage the loosening of sputum.
- Better tolerated by the woman but the circuit can be unwieldy and complex to set up – anaesthetic assistants can be very useful in setting up this equipment on the labour ward.
- The flow-meter selects the oxygen concentration delivered from 28%–90%

Nebulisers for use in the treatment of bronchospasm
- A flow rate of 6 to 8 L/min of oxygen or air is required to nebulise the liquid into small droplets for inhalation.
- Salbutamol (2.5 mg) and ipratropium bromide (500 **micrograms**) may be combined to make up to 4.5 mL.
- Nebulising time is approximately 5–10 minutes.
- Side effects include tachycardia, and eye irritation (if facemask is used).

Prescribing oxygen

When prescribing oxygen, you should include:
- Whether oxygen saturation monitoring is required
- The desired target oxygen saturations (usually 94–98%)
- Whether humidification is required
- The duration for which the oxygen will be required
- The oxygen type of delivery device to be used

In an emergency when oxygen is required, it can be initiated before the prescription is completed.

Non-invasive ventilation

CPAP (continuous positive airway pressure)
- A type of ventilation in which the woman breathes out against a high flow of gas (e.g. oxygen)
- Helps prevent airway collapse by 'splinting' open the smaller airways (adults achieve a similar effect by breathing with tightly pursed lips; neonates achieve this through grunting)
- Can be delivered using a tight-fitting mask, or by using specialised nasal cannulae which are often better tolerated but may mean that the administration is less accurate
- Is often described in terms of the pressure the woman breathes against (e.g. 5 cmH$_2$O) as

well as the inspired oxygen concentration

- Typically increases the level of oxygen in arterial blood (PaO_2), but does not affect the level the level of carbon dioxide in arterial blood ($PaCO_2$)
- Can be a useful treatment of severe hypoxaemia (in type I respiratory failure: i.e. where oxygenation is low, but the effort of breathing is adequate), and of pulmonary oedema
- Can be used in an attempt to avoid invasive ventilation (i.e. intubation and ventilation)

BiPAP (bi-level positive airway pressure)

- A type of ventilation in which the ventilator pushes air at a higher pressure into the lungs during inspiration (the inspiratory pressure), and a lower pressure against which the woman breathes during expiration (the expiratory pressure)
- Helps increase the tidal volume (the volume of each breath), thereby increasing the minute ventilation (the volume breathed each minute) and hence reducing $PaCO_2$
- Is typically described using the inspiratory pressure over the expiratory pressure (e.g. 12/5 cmH_2O) as well as the inspired oxygen concentration (e.g. 50% oxygen)
- Typically improves the PaO_2 as well as the $PaCO_2$
- Can be a useful treatment of type II respiratory failure (where ventilation is inadequate, and the $PaCO_2$ is raised)
- Can be used to avoid invasive ventilation (i.e. intubation and ventilation)

Complications of oxygen administration

- Oxygen concentrations will be affected with all delivery systems if not fitted correctly or if delivery tubing becomes kinked or ports are obstructed
- Oxygen is an ignition hazard. To reduce the risks of fire, valves on oxygen cylinders should be closed when not in use.
- It is important to check that the prescribed amount of oxygen is being dispensed, particularly when using an oxygen cylinder, as the green indicator on the flow meter showing that the cylinder is full, can be misinterpreted as an indicator of active flow. All relevant clinical staff should receive training in the safe use of oxygen cylinders. (1).
- Oxygen may cause atelectasis and lung tissue damage at high concentration (e.g. > 60% oxygen for prolonged periods)
- Respiratory depression is possible in a minority of women with very severe chronic obstructive pulmonary disease (COPD) if high concentrations of oxygen are administered ('CO_2 retainers').

Arterial blood gases

> **Blood gases normal values:**
> - pH: 7.35 to 7.45
> - PaO_2: > 10 kPa breathing room air
> - $PaCO_2$: 4.7 to 6.0 kPa
> - HCO_3^- : 22 to 26 mmol/L
> - Base excess: -2 to +2 mmol/L

Arterial blood gas samples can be taken from an arterial line (for more information see **Section 6**), or as a one-off specimen using a needle and syringe from the artery (although this is painful and if more than one sample is needed an arterial line should be considered). Depending on the setup of the analyser, other information may also be given including a haemoglobin, some electrolytes, glucose level and a lactate level.

The 5-step approach to arterial blood gas interpretation

1. What is the condition of the woman?

- This will provide valuable clues to help with interpretation of the results

2. Determine the pH (or H^+ concentration)

- Is the woman acidaemic? pH < 7.35 (H^+ > 45 nmol/L)
- Is the woman alkalaemic? pH > 7.45 (H^+ < 35 nmol/L)
- Normal pH is 7.35 to 7.45

3. Determine the respiratory component

- $PaCO_2$ > 6.0 kPa (45 mmHg)
  - this is a 'respiratory acidosis'
  - caused by <u>hypo</u>ventilation, e.g. from lung disease or inadequate respiratory effort
  - or (rarely) respiratory compensation for a metabolic alkalosis
- $PaCO_2$ < 4.7 kPa (35 mmHg)
  - usually caused by hyperventilation
  - can be respiratory compensation for a metabolic acidosis
  - rarely represents a primary respiratory alkalosis

4. Determine the metabolic component

- HCO_3^- < 22 mmol/L (equivalent to base excess < -2 mmol/L)
    - this is a 'metabolic acidosis'
    - or (rarely) renal compensation for a respiratory alkalosis
- HCO_3^- > 26 mmol/L (equivalent to base excess > +2 mmol/L)
    - renal compensation for a respiratory acidosis (long-term compensation)
    - or (rarely) metabolic alkalosis
- Some clinicians prefer to use the base excess (or deficit) instead of the HCO_3^-, and as the changes in these values mirror each other, either can be used.
- The normal base excess is zero (normal range -2 to +2 mmol/L)
- It can be useful to examine the bicarbonate and/or base excess in the context of the serum lactate, as a raised lactate (> 2 mmol/L) is another biomarker of reduced tissue perfusion.

5. Assess oxygenation

- Is the woman hypoxaemic?
- The PaO_2 should be > 10 kPa (75mmHg) on air, and about 10 kPa less than the percentage inspired oxygen concentration (e.g. the PaO_2 should be approximately 30 kPa if a woman is breathing 40% oxygen)

All of the above information can then be drawn together to produce a final diagnosis of the primary disturbance, any degree of compensation and any indication of disturbance of oxygenation.

Most critically ill women tend to have an acidosis: either metabolic acidosis due to poor tissue perfusion, respiratory acidosis due to respiratory failure, or a mixed metabolic and respiratory acidosis.

Finally, any other measurements displayed on the blood gas result should be reviewed and interpreted in correlation with the woman's clinical condition.

Management of critically ill pregnant and postpartum women with abnormal blood gases

Metabolic acidosis

Metabolic acidosis in critically ill women is often due to lactic acidosis. This occurs when the body's tissues do not have enough oxygen to meet their needs; typically, due to poor tissue perfusion. Oxygen delivery can be improved by:

- Increasing the inspired oxygen concentration (which is why all critical ill women require supplemental oxygen)

- Increasing the cardiac output, such as through increasing the circulating volume by giving a fluid challenge of 250–500 mL crystalloid. Inotropes and/or vasopressors may be required to further improve organ perfusion if fluid challenges are insufficient: this may be an indication for transfer to Level 3 care.

- Raising the haemoglobin concentration if the woman is anaemic.

Respiratory acidosis

A raised $PaCO_2$ in a previously well woman that is spontaneously breathing (i.e. not on a ventilator) is a worrying sign. Drugs, such as opioids, or sedation, may have reduced the woman's respiratory effort. A raised $PaCO_2$ also occurs when a woman's respiratory reserve is exhausted and she is no longer able to breathe effectively: this is a form of respiratory failure.

Respiratory failure with a raised $PaCO_2$ is called type II respiratory failure and requires timely management. An anaesthetist should be contacted as the woman may require respiratory support (such as bi-level positive airway pressure – BiPAP, or invasive respiratory support, i.e. intubation and ventilation).

Hypoxaemia

A reduced arterial oxygen level should be managed with supplemental oxygen therapy, as described above. Remember that the PaO_2 needs to be considered in the context of the oxygen concentration that the woman is receiving (i.e. a PaO_2 of 12 kPa is acceptable if the woman is breathing room air but would represent significant hypoxaemia if the woman is breathing high-flow oxygen). A reduced PaO_2 with a normal or low $PaCO_2$ is termed type I respiratory failure.

If simple oxygen therapy alone is unable to improve the arterial oxygen saturation to acceptable levels (i.e. $\geq 95\%$), the woman should be discussed with the critical care team as more specialised respiratory support such as continuous positive airway pressure (CPAP) may be required. Very severe hypoxaemia may require invasive respiratory support, i.e. intubation and ventilation.

Pregnant – or recently pregnant – women with life-threatening respiratory failure, which persists despite optimal invasive ventilation on the intensive care unit, should be considered for extracorporeal membrane oxygenation (ECMO) (2). This highly specialised form of respiratory support, similar to cardiopulmonary bypass, can be life-saving in the most severe cases of respiratory failure, however is available in very few adult centres in the UK.

References

1. NHS Patient Safety Alert, January 2018:
    https://improvement.nhs.uk/documents/2206/Patient_Safety_Alert_-
    _Failure_to_open_oxygen_cylinders.pdf. Accessed 8 June 2018.

2. Knight M, Nair M, Tuffnell D, Kenyon S, Shakespeare J, Brocklehurst P, et al., editors. Saving Lives, Improving Mothers' Care. 2016 pp. 1–120.

Section 5: ECGs and rhythm recognition

Key Learning Point
▪ ECGs and cardiac rhythms should always be interpreted in the context of the woman's clinical condition

Cardiac changes in pregnancy

To achieve the increased cardiac output that is required for pregnancy the resting heart rate is higher, and at term the maternal heart rate is often between 80 and 100 beats per minute. Bradycardia during pregnancy, a heart rate less than 60 beats per minute, is unusual and should be investigated.

The electrocardiogram (ECG) measures the electrical activity through the heart. The ECG in a pregnant woman may be normal or may display any of the following variables due to the physiological changes of pregnancy.

Normal ECG changes that can be present in pregnancy:

- Relative tachycardia
- Atrial and ventricular ectopic beats
- Left axis shift
- ST depression (of less than 2 mm)
- T wave inversion in the inferolateral leads (II, III, aVF, and V5 and V6)

ECG

An ECG is usually performed using 3 or 12 'leads'.

A 3-lead ECG can be used for continuous cardiac monitoring in theatre, post-operatively and in the critically ill pregnant or postpartum woman. The 3-lead ECG provides continuous information on the cardiac rate and rhythm.

A 12-lead ECG provides more detail on the cardiac electrical activity. Ten electrodes are placed on the surface of the chest and on the woman's limbs. The overall magnitude of the heart's electrical potential is then measured from 12 different angles ('leads') and is recorded over 10 seconds. A

12-lead ECG not only provides information about the rate and rhythm of the heart but also reflects the size and position of the heart chambers and the presence of any damage to the heart's muscle cells or conduction system.

Lead Placement

- 3-lead ECG electrode placement
  - RA (Right Arm) – red (often placed on the right shoulder)
  - LA (Left Arm) – yellow (often placed on the left shoulder)
    LL (Left Leg) – green (often placed on the left lower chest)
- 3-lead ECG leads
  - Lead I: looks at the heart's electrical signal in a line from the red to the yellow electrode, i.e. across the top of the chest
  - Lead II: looks at the heart's electrical signal in a line from the red to the green electrode. This follows the main electrical signals travelling through the heart, and is therefore usually the best lead to examine the heart rhythm
  - Lead III: looks at the heart's electrical signal in a line from the yellow to the green electrode, i.e. down the lateral side of the chest
- 12-lead ECG
  - Standard limb leads
    - Lead I (as above)
    - Lead II (as above)
    - Lead III (as above)
  - Chest Electrode Placement
    - V1: 4th intercostal space right of the sternum.
    - V2: 4th intercostal space Left of the sternum.
    - V3: Between leads V2 and V4.
    - V4: 5th intercostal space mid-clavicular line.
    - V5: Level with V4 at left anterior axillary line.
    - V6: Level with V5 at left mid-axillary line.
  - Augmented limb leads:
    - aVR: from the cenre of the heart to the red electrode
    - aVL: from the centre of the heart to the yellow electrode
    - aVF: from the centre of the heart to the green electrode (i.e. straight down the body)

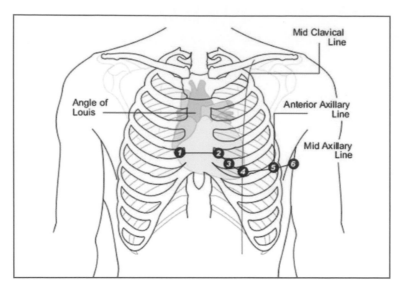

The 12-lead ECG allows a more detailed examination of the electrical activity of the heart, providing evidence of ischaemia or myocardial infarction, and which part of the heart is affected by these conditions.

Interpreting the ECG:

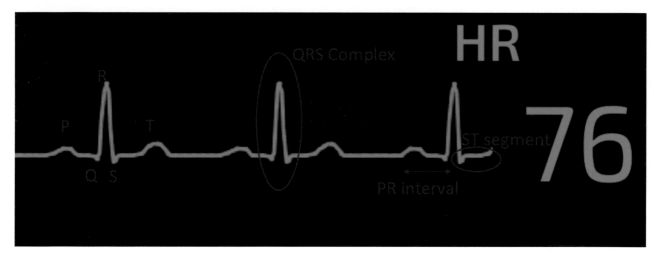

Rate:

This is the number of heart beats per minute. The normal heart rate is 60–100; a heart rate faster than 100 beats per minute (bpm) is termed tachycardia and less than 60 bpm is termed bradycardia.

Rhythm:

Sinus rhythm is the normal heart rhythm. In sinus rhythm the heart rate is regular, there are normal P waves, and each P wave is followed by a QRS complex.

Other heart rhythms include:

- o Atrial fibrillation (AF) – an irregular heart rhythm, without distinguishable P waves

- Atrial flutter – a regular heart rhythm where P waves are replaced by saw-toothed flutter waves
- Ventricular fibrillation (VF) – an irregular heart rhythm without any organised electrical activity. In VF there are no synchronised signals making the heart contract, and so the patient will be in cardiac arrest

An overview of the main heart rhythms is covered in more detail later in this section.

P wave:

This is the electrical activity from the depolarisation (wave of electrical current) of the atria and is triggered by pacemaker cells in the sinoatrial (SA) node in health. P waves usually indicate that the atria are contracting normally.

PR interval:

This is the time between the start of the P wave until the start of the QRS complex. It usually lasts 120–200 ms (3–5 small squares on a 12-lead ECG). The PR interval may be prolonged in various types of heart block.

QRS complex:

This is the electrical activity from the depolarisation of the ventricles and is triggered, in health, by pacemaker cells in the atrioventricular (AV) node in response to the arrival of a P wave from the atria. The QRS complex is usually 'narrow complex' (i.e. less than 120 ms: 3 small squares on the 12-lead ECG). If the QRS complex lasts longer than 120 ms, these are 'broad complex' rhythms; this usually signifies that either:

- There is a delay in the electrical signals passing through the ventricles (e.g. left and right bundle branch blocks)
- The ventricles' electrical signals are not being generated from the AV node (e.g. ventricular tachycardia, some types of heart block)

ST segment:

Usually, in the section between the QRS complex and the T wave, the ECG returns to baseline. If the ST segment is below the baseline, this may represent myocardial ischaemia. If the ST segment is elevated above the baseline, this may indicate myocardial infarction (STEMI = ST elevation myocardial infarction); see the 'myocardial infarction' section below.

T wave:

The T wave represents the repolarisation of the ventricles, i.e. their return to their baseline electrical activity. T waves are usually shaped like a small hill and rise above the baseline in most leads of the 12-lead ECG. T waves can be inverted in certain conditions (e.g. myocardial ischaemia, subarachnoid haemorrhage, pulmonary embolus, in patients with a previous myocardial infarction). T waves are tall and tented (triangular) in severe hyperkalaemia (see **Section 3**).

When looking at an ECG the following questions should be answered:

- What is the rate?
- Are the complexes regular?
- Is the P wave present?
- Is each P wave followed by a QRS complex?
- Are the QRS complexes widened/distorted?
- Are the ST segments above or below the baseline?
- Are the T waves normal?

When assessing the woman in the context of her ECG, first ask:

- **'How is the woman?'**
    - If she is collapsed, unresponsive and not breathing normally then the woman should be treated as if she is in cardiac arrest. Call for help (2222), displace the uterus and begin CPR (see **Figure 5.1**)
    - If she is compromised, call for help and assess her using an ABCDE approach. ECG abnormalities leading to severe compromise often will require treatment with sedation/general anaesthesia and synchronised electric shock (electrical pacing in bradycardia, DC cardioversion in tachycardia)

Sinus rhythm

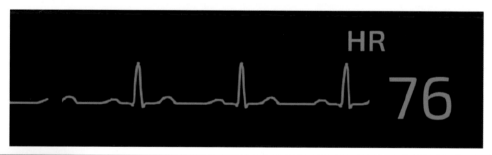

Rate	60–100 bpm
Rhythm	Regular
P-wave	Before each QRS
PR interval	Normal (< 5 small squares = 200 ms)
QRS duration	Normal (i.e. narrow complex, < 3 small squares = 120 ms)
Comment	Indicates the electrical signal originates in the sinus node and travels normally through the heart.

This is the normal heart rhythm in health.

Sinus bradycardia

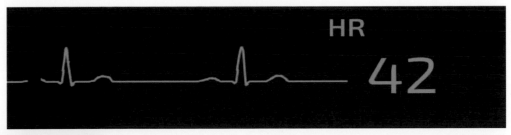

Rate	< 60 bpm
Rhythm	Regular
P-wave	Before each QRS
PR interval	Normal (< 5 small squares = 200 ms)
QRS duration	Normal (i.e. narrow complex, < 3 small squares = 120 ms)
Comment	In a healthy athletic person this may be 'normal' Anything that increases vagal tone, e.g. drug abuse, hypoglycaemia, cervical stimulation, brain injury with raised intracranial pressure (ICP).

A heart rate below 60 is termed bradycardia; this can be normal in healthy athletic people, although is less commonly seen in pregnant women due to the physiological changes of pregnancy. A heart rate below 40 is severe bradycardia and is rarely normal. Bradycardia can be caused by damage to the heart's electrical pathways, by electrolyte imbalance, and by some drugs (such as β-blockers and anti-arrhythmics). The woman may be asymptomatic, although they might be aware of their heart beating slowly; or they may be compromised with light-headedness, chest pain or collapse.

Management of bradycardia:

How is the woman? If the woman is <u>well</u>, with a heart rate between 40 and 60 beats per minute, no specific treatment is indicated apart from continued observation and identifying the cause.

If the woman is <u>compromised</u> (SBP < 90 mmHg, clammy, impaired consciousness, chest pain, unconscious):

- o Call for help (2222)
- o A: Ensure airway is patent
- o B: High flow oxygen, continuous SpO_2 monitoring
- o C: Left lateral (if pregnant), IV access, continuous ECG monitoring, 12-lead ECG. Continuous CTG monitoring if antenatal/in labour
- o Treat any obvious cause

- o Anaesthetist or critical care team will evaluate the potential need for drugs (atropine, isoprenaline, adrenaline) or electrical pacing

Sinus tachycardia

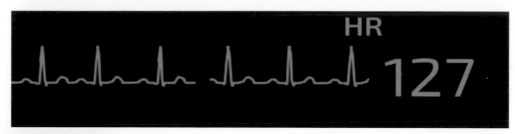

Rate	> 100 bpm
Rhythm	Regular
P-wave	Before each QRS
PR interval	Normal (< 5 small squares = 200 ms)
QRS duration	Normal (i.e. narrow complex, < 3 small squares = 120 ms)
Comment	Caused by exercise, shock, stress, illness, fever, anxiety, dehydration, sepsis, pain, drugs, anaemia.

Sinus tachycardia is a normal response to exertion (e.g. exercise, labour), pain, anxiety, stress and certain medications (e.g. terbutaline, salbutamol or other β_2-agonists). Abnormal conditions such as haemorrhage, sepsis, pulmonary embolism, electrolyte abnormalities and hyperthyroidism can also cause sinus tachycardia. A sustained heart rate above 120 bpm is unusual and should prompt a medical review.

Management of sinus tachycardia:

How is the woman? If the woman is <u>well</u>, and the cause is obvious and not harmful, no further action may be required apart from continued observation and consideration of the cause.

If the woman is <u>compromised</u> (HR > 120 bpm, SBP 90 mmHg, clammy, impaired consciousness, chest pain, unconscious):

- o Call for obstetric/medical help (2222 if severely compromised)
- o A: Ensure airway is patent
- o B: Consider high flow oxygen and continuous SpO_2 monitoring
- o C: Left lateral (if pregnant), IV access, consider continuous ECG monitoring and 12-lead ECG. Consider continuous CTG if antenatal/in labour
- o Management should be aimed at identifying and treating the cause

Supraventricular tachycardia (SVT) – abnormal

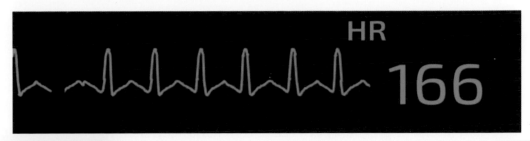

Rate	140–220 bpm
Rhythm	Regular
P-wave	Often hidden in the T-wave
PR interval	Depends on the site of the supraventricular pacemaker
QRS duration	Usually normal (i.e.narrow complex, < 3 small squares = 120 ms)
Comment	Typically caused by drugs or abnormal conduction pathways.

SVT can be triggered by caffeine, alcohol, drugs (e.g. medication such as β_2-agonists like terbutaline or salbutamol, or illicit drugs such as cocaine) or electrolyte abnormalities; it can also be caused by structural abnormalities within the heart's electrical pathways.

Many women may be well, some may even have had SVT before; however, some may be severely compromised. The woman may say they feel palpitations (being aware that her heart is beating fast), short of breath or lightheaded; she may even complain of chest pain.

Management of SVT:

How is the woman? If the woman is <u>well</u>:

- o Call for medical/obstetric help
- o Consider IV access
- o Continuous ECG monitoring
- o Continuous CTG monitoring if antenatal/in labour
- o Treat any obvious cause (e.g. electrolyte abnormalities)
- o Consider vagal manoeuvres:
  - Ask the woman to blow into the barrel of a 10 mL syringe
  - Carotid sinus massage (if you are trained to do so)
- o Consider chemical cardioversion:
  - Some women will have their own prescribed oral anti-arrhythmics (e.g. verapamil)
  - Adenosine (6 mg, 12 mg, 12 mg): requires IV access, resuscitation equipment available. May cause chest discomfort/feeling unwell

If the woman is <u>compromised</u> (SBP < 90 mmHg, clammy, impaired consciousness, chest pain, unconscious):

- o Call for help (2222)
- o A: Ensure airway is patent
- o B: High flow oxygen, continuous SpO$_2$ monitoring
- o C: Left lateral (if pregnant), IV access, continuous ECG monitoring, 12-lead ECG
  Continuous CTG monitoring if antenatal/in labour
- o Treat any obvious cause (e.g. electrolyte abnormalities)
- o Anaesthetist or critical care team needed to allow synchronised DC cardioversion under sedation/general anaesthesia

Once the woman has been successfully reverted to sinus rhythm:

- 12-lead ECG to confirm the successful cardioversion
- Refer to cardiology for follow-up

If the cardioversion is unsuccessful, refer to cardiology for expert opinion.

Atrial fibrillation – abnormal

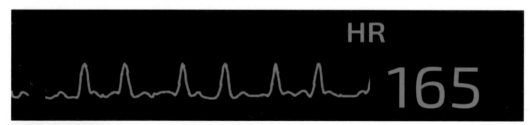

Rate	100–160 bpm
Rhythm	Irregularly irregular
P-wave	Not distinguishable
PR interval	Not measurable
QRS duration	Usually normal (i.e. narrow complex, < 3 small squares = 120 ms)
Comment	Multiple sites in the atria generate electrical impulses, causing irregular conduction to the ventricles (an irregular rhythm can be felt when palpating a pulse). Caused by valve diseases, sick sinus syndrome, pericarditis, lung disease and congenital heart defects, electrolyte disturbances, or can be idiopathic.

In atrial fibrillation (AF) the random nature of the electrical activity in the atria means that they do not contract, and also uncoordinated signals are sent via the AV node to the ventricles. As a result, the heart rate is irregular, and the contraction of the heart may be reduced as blood does not reach the ventricles efficiently. Combined with the potential for significant tachycardia (so-called 'fast AF'), AF sometimes leads to significant cardiovascular compromise.

The lack of atrial contraction also means that blood can stagnate within the heart, risking the formation of atrial thrombus (blood clot), which can embolise causing a stroke or other vascular occlusion such as ischaemic bowel.

Atrial fibrillation can be caused by damage to the heart's electrical pathways, by electrolyte abnormalities (e.g. low K^+ or low Mg^{2+}), hyperthyroidism, stimulants (such as medications, caffeine and alcohol) and lung diseases. AF can occur periodically ('paroxysmal' AF), as a one-off episode, or it can be chronic. Many women with AF will feel well and will just be aware of their irregular heartbeat; however, some may be compromised with light-headedness, breathlessness, chest pain or collapse.

Management of atrial fibrillation (AF):

How is the woman?

If the woman is <u>well</u> and not compromised, it is important to determine the onset of the AF. AF lasting longer than 48 hours leads to a significant risk of thrombus formation; any attempt to cardiovert (i.e. convert back to sinus rhythm using drugs or electricity) risks the thrombus being released into the circulation as an embolus, causing a stroke or other vascular occlusion. Therefore, anticoagulation and rate-control are the priorities. If the onset of AF is under 48 hours, then cardioversion can be considered.

The management of stable AF is complex, and advice should be sought from a cardiologist or physician. In the meantime, treat any obvious cause (e.g. electrolyte abnormalities).

If the woman is <u>compromised</u> (SBP < 90 mmHg, clammy, impaired consciousness, chest pain, unconscious):

- Call for help (2222)
- A: Ensure airway is patent
- B: High flow oxygen, continuous SpO_2 monitoring
- C: Left lateral (if pregnant), IV access, continuous ECG monitoring, 12-lead ECG. Continuous CTG monitoring if antenatal/in labour
- Treat any obvious cause (e.g. electrolyte abnormalities)

o Anaesthetist or critical care team needed to allow synchronised DC cardioversion under sedation/general anaesthesia

Once the woman has been successfully reverted to sinus rhythm:

- 12-lead ECG to confirm the successful cardioversion
- Refer to cardiology for follow-up

If the cardioversion is unsuccessful, refer to cardiology for expert opinion.

Atrial flutter – abnormal

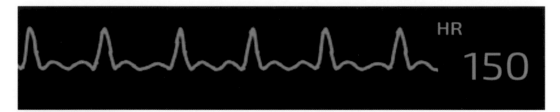

Rate	QRS rate often around 150 bpm
Rhythm	Regular
P-wave	No true P-wave, instead multiple F- (flutter) waves at a rate of 300bpm, usually a ratio of 2:1 sometimes 3:1 transmission to the ventricle (2–3 flutter waves for every QRS)
PR interval	Not measurable
QRS duration	Usually normal (i.e. narrow complex, < 3 small squares = 120 ms)
Comment	Abnormal tissue in the atria generating the rapid heart rate. The atrioventricular node is not involved. Caused by mitral valve disease, pulmonary embolism, thoracic surgery, hypoxia, electrolyte disturbances and hypocalcaemia.

Management of atrial flutter:

The immediate management of the pregnant woman with atrial flutter may follow the same pathway as atrial fibrillation (see previous), but the subsequent management may be different and requires specialist input.

Ventricular tachycardia (VT) - abnormal

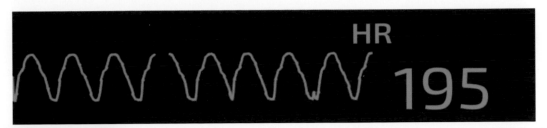

Rate	180–200 bpm
Rhythm	Regular
P-wave	Not seen
PR interval	Not measurable
QRS duration	Prolonged (> 3 small squares)
Comment	Caused by abnormal electrical activity in the ventricles which generates a rapid, irregular heart rhythm with a poor cardiac output.
	Some women will have a pulse and be responsive; they are likely to be compromised and are at risk of deteriorating into cardiac arrest.
	Some women will be unresponsive with no pulse; they are in cardiac arrest. They require CPR and early defibrillation.

Management of ventricular tachycardia (VT):

How is the woman?

If she is <u>collapsed</u>, is not breathing and has no pulse, this is cardiac arrest:

- o Call for help (2222)
- o Left uterine displacement (if pregnant)
- o Begin CPR (30:2)
- o Early defibrillation (AED or manual defibrillator) is essential
- o Follow ALS algorithm (see **Figure 5.1**)
- o Consider the four **Hs** and four **Ts** (see **Box 5.1**)

If she <u>has a pulse but is compromised</u> (SBP < 90 mmHg, clammy, impaired consciousness, chest pain, unconscious):

- o Call for help (2222)
- o A: Ensure airway is patent
- o B: High flow oxygen, continuous SpO_2 monitoring

- C: Left lateral (if pregnant), IV access, continuous ECG monitoring, 12-lead ECG. Continuous CTG monitoring if antenatal/in labour
- Treat any obvious cause (e.g. electrolyte abnormalities)
- Anaesthetist or critical care team needed to allow *synchronised* DC cardioversion under sedation/general anaesthesia

Once the woman has been successfully reverted to sinus rhythm:

- 12-lead ECG to confirm the successful cardioversion
- Refer to cardiology for follow-up
- If woman is pregnant, assess fetal well-being

If the cardioversion is unsuccessful, refer to cardiology for expert opinion.

If she is <u>responsive and not compromised</u>:

- Call for medical/obstetric help (consider 2222)
- A: Ensure airway is patent
- B: High flow oxygen, continuous SpO$_2$ monitoring
- C: Left lateral (if pregnant), IV access, continuous ECG monitoring, 12-lead ECG. Continuous CTG monitoring if antenatal/in labour
- Treat any obvious cause (e.g. electrolyte abnormalities)
- Anaesthetist and cardiologist/physician needed to consider the need for chemical cardioversion (e.g. with amiodarone)

Once the woman has been successfully reverted to sinus rhythm:

- 12-lead ECG to confirm the successful cardioversion
- Refer to cardiology for follow-up

If the cardioversion is unsuccessful, refer to cardiology for expert opinion.

Ventricular fibrillation (VF) – abnormal

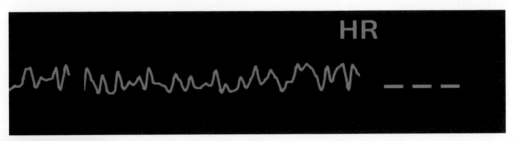

Rate	> 300 but disorganised
Rhythm	Irregular
P-wave	Not seen
PR interval	Not measurable
QRS duration	Not recognisable
Comment	VF is caused by disorganised electrical signals which stimulate the ventricles causing them to quiver ineffectively. This heart rhythm is incompatible with a cardiac output, and therefore is a cardiac arrest rhythm. It requires CPR and early defibrillation.

Management of ventricular fibrillation (VF):

How is the woman? If she is collapsed, is not breathing and has no pulse, this is cardiac arrest:

- o Call for help (2222)
- o Left uterine displacement (if pregnant)
- o Begin CPR
- o Early defibrillation (AED or manual defibrillator) is essential
- o Follow ALS algorithm (see **Figure 5.1**)
- o Consider the four **Hs** and four **Ts**

Figure 5.1 Advanced Life Support (ALS) algorithm (based on Resuscitation Council (UK) Guidelines, 2015 (1)

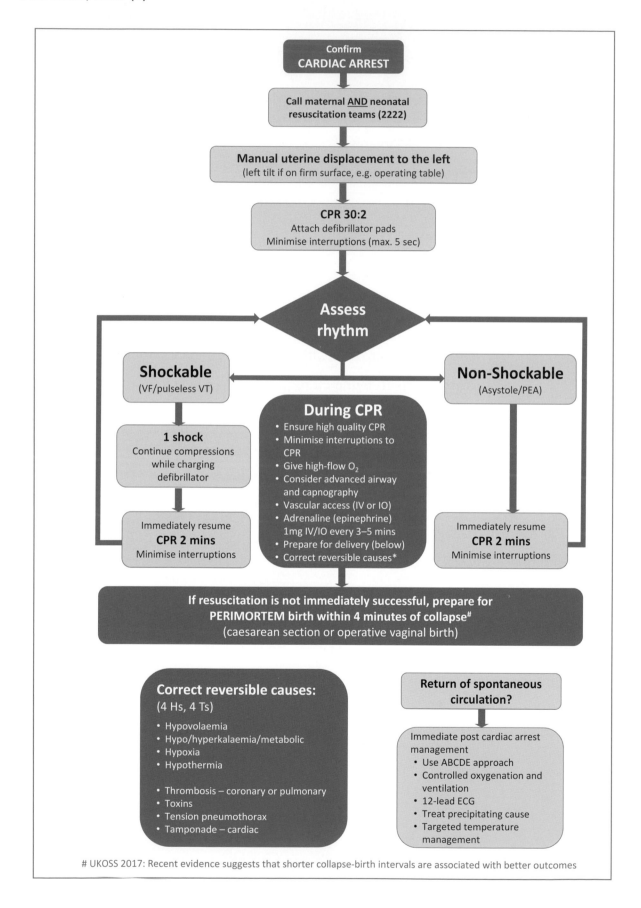

Asystole – abnormal

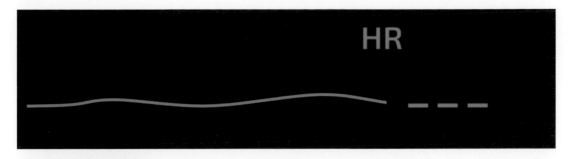

Rate	0 bpm
Rhythm	Flat trace with an undulating baseline
P-wave	None
PR interval	None
QRS duration	None
Comment	Asystole means that the heart is not generating any electrical activity, and the woman is therefore in cardiac arrest. Asystole has the worst prognosis of all the cardiac arrest rhythms.

Management of asystole:

How is the woman? If she is collapsed, is not breathing and has no pulse, this is cardiac arrest:

- o   Call for help (2222)
- o   Left uterine displacement
- o   Begin CPR
- o   Follow ALS algorithm (see **Figure 5.1**)
- o   Consider the four **Hs** and four **Ts** (see **Box 5.1**)

Myocardial infarction (MI) – abnormal

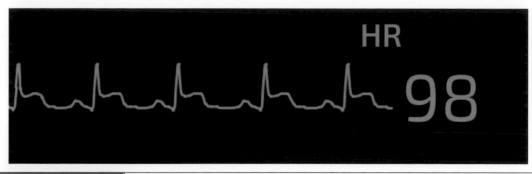

Rate	Not specific
Rhythm	Regular or irregular
P-wave	Typically normal
PR interval	Typically normal
QRS duration	Normal or slightly prolonged
Comment	NSTEMI (non-ST-elevation MI) is diagnosed from history, ECG changes and biochemical markers (e.g. troponin). STEMI (ST-elevation MI) can be diagnosed from history and ECG changes alone.

Further information on myocardial infarction and its management can be found in **Section 7**.

Myocardial infarction is caused by a blockage to the coronary arteries that perfuse the heart muscle and its conducting tissue. If caught early, the blockage can be cleared and permanent cardiac damage can be avoided. Myocardial infarction is therefore a medical emergency. In addition, myocardial infarction can also lead to arrhythmias including cardiac arrest rhythms such as VF and VT.

The woman will often complain of chest pain or tightness; this is typically described as 'squeezing' or 'vice-like', and may radiate to the neck, jaw, left arm or epigastrium. Any woman presenting with chest pain needs urgent evaluation, and investigation.

The coronary arteries can be unblocked either physically or through the use of medication:

Physically: PCI – percutaneous coronary intervention

- o Performed by an interventional cardiologist in specialist centres
- o Involves taking x-ray pictures of the blocked arteries (angiogram)
- o A deflated balloon is then passed into the blocked artery
- o The balloon is inflated to open up the artery (angioplasty)
- o A stent can be left to keep the artery open

- o The woman will then require potent antiplatelet drugs to keep the stent patent for subsequent months; this will put her at increased risk of bleeding

- o This is the most effective means of treating MI

Medically: thrombolysis

- o Can be performed by any medical professional who has been trained to do so

- o Involves the injection of potent drugs that dissolve blood clots (thrombolytics)

- o The woman will be at high risk of bleeding over the subsequent few hours

- o Thrombolysis is slightly less effective means of treating MI, however thrombolysis might be a more-timely intervention depending on the location of the woman

The management of suspected MI is multifactorial and requires the urgent input of a cardiologist, hence the aphorism 'time is muscle'.

Management of suspected myocardial infarction (MI):

How is the woman?

If she is <u>collapsed</u>, unresponsive and not breathing normally, then the woman should be treated as if she is in cardiac arrest:

- o Call for help (2222)

- o Left uterine displacement (if pregnant)

- o Begin CPR

- o Follow ALS algorithm (see **Figure 5.1**)

If she <u>has a pulse</u>:

- o Call for help (consider 2222)

- o A: Ensure airway is patent

- o B: High flow oxygen if SpO_2 < 94%, continuous SpO_2 monitoring

- o C: IV access, continuous ECG monitoring, 12-lead ECG. Continuous CTG monitoring if antenatal/in labour

- o GTN sublingual spray (only if SBP > 90 mmHg)

- o Give aspirin 300 mg orally (dispersible aspirin or chewed tablet has more rapid absorption)

- o Offer analgesia (e.g. morphine 3–5 mg IV)

- o Contact cardiologist to determine definitive management

Pulseless Electrical Activity (PEA)

- o Occurs when ECG activity observed on the electrocardiogram (ECG) does not produce a perfusing rhythm. PEA can come in many different forms.
  - o Sinus rhythm, tachycardia, and bradycardia can all be seen with PEA.

Management of PEA:

How is the woman? If she is <u>collapsed</u>, unresponsive and not breathing normally, she should be treated as if she is in cardiac arrest:

- o Call for help (2222)
- o Left uterine displacement
- o Begin CPR
- o Follow ALS algorithm (see **Figure 5.1**)
- o Consider the four **Hs** and four **Ts** (see **Box 5.1**):

Box 5.1 The four Hs and four Ts (potentially reversible causes of cardiac arrest)

- Hypoxia
- Hypovolaemia
- Hypo-/hyperkalaemia/metabolic
- Hypothermia

- Thrombosis – coronary or pulmonary
- Tamponade – cardiac
- Toxins
- Tension pneumothorax

For more information concerning the management of maternal collapse, and basic and advanced life support we recommend reading the relevant modules in the PROMPT Course Manual (Third Edition).

References

1   Available from https://www.resus.org.uk/resuscitation-guidelines/adult-advanced-life-support/#algorithm

2   Beckett VA, Knight M, Sharpe P. The CAPS Study: incidence, management and outcomes of cardiac arrest in pregnancy in the UK: a prospective, descriptive study. BJOG: Br J Obstet Gynaecol. 2017 Feb 24;124(9):1374–81.

Section 6: Invasive monitoring

Arterial Lines

Arterial lines are cannulae placed in one of the peripheral arteries. They are used to:

- Provide continuous (i.e. beat-to-beat) monitoring of the blood pressure
- Acquire arterial blood gases or other blood samples

The tubing of the arterial line is easily identifiable due to its red colour (representing arterial blood)

Figure 6.1 Example of an arterial line cannula (note the red markings to distinguish it from an intravenous cannula)

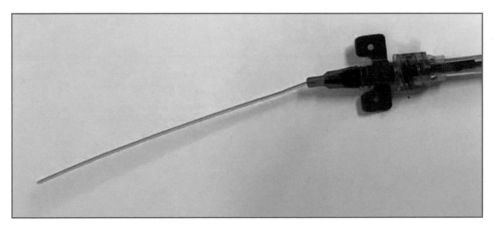

Arterial line insertion

- Arterial lines can be placed into:
    - Radial artery at the wrist (this is the most common site)
    - Brachial artery in the antecubital fossa
    - Dorsalis pedis artery on the back of the foot
    - Femoral artery at the groin

Equipment required for arterial line insertion and monitoring

- Arterial cannula
- Many hospitals have a sterile pre-packed kit containing the necessary disposables:
    - Sterile gauze
    - 2 mL and 5 mL syringes
    - Needle for injection
    - Sterile drape
    - Occlusive transparent dressings
    - Sterile gloves
- Local anaesthetic (usually 5 to 10 mL 1% lidocaine)
- Transducer set run through from a 500 mL 0.9% saline/heparinised saline bag
- Pressure bag over the 500 mL bag of saline/heparinised saline inflated to 300 mmHg
- Transducer cable
- Monitor

Potential complications

- Haemorrhage:
    - The arterial system is under high pressure and therefore the major risk of an arterial line is haemorrhage; it is therefore imperative that all connectors are securely fastened and all taps are closed.
- Ischaemia distal to the arterial line:
    - No drugs or medication should <u>ever</u> be injected into an arterial line. The arteries gradually decrease in size and become arterioles and then capillaries. Particles contained in drugs can become lodged in the capillary system which can lead to distal ischaemia (e.g. of the hand, finger and thumb).
    - Arterial damage can also cause distal ischaemia
- Incorrect position of catheter
- "Tissue-ing" of the cannula
- Bleeding from the puncture site
- Infection
- Arterial damage
- Haematoma

> **Red caps and/or tubing should be used on arterial lines (and nowhere else)**
>
> **Do <u>not</u> let ANYONE inject into an arterial line**
>
> **Only a trained doctor or nurse/midwife should take the sample and flush the arterial line after sampling**

Taking an invasive blood pressure measurement

- Explain to the woman what you are going to do
- Align the transducer with the fifth intercostal space in the mid-axillary line (the surface landmark of the right atrium of the heart)
- Check that the flush system is pressurised to 300 mmHg (e.g. by inflating the pressure bag over the 500mL bag of saline/heparinised saline and ensuring the pressure is in the 'green zone') and flush the line to check its patency
- 'Zero' the transducer
  - This sets the monitor so that its 0 mmHg reading is at the current ambient atmospheric pressure
- Check the arterial line trace
- Document the reading and report any changes or abnormalities

It is imperative that the bag of fluids used for flushing the set is double checked at the time it is put up and at every shift change to ensure it is compliant with local protocol. Most units use either 0.9% saline or a heparinised saline. Inadvertent use of bags containing glucose can lead to complications in the management of blood sugars. This is a particular problem if the woman is sedated on an intensive care unit and is receiving insulin as blood gases can give a falsely high blood sugar measurement, resulting in more insulin administration and the development of hypoglycaemia (1).

Figure 6.2 Arterial line set components

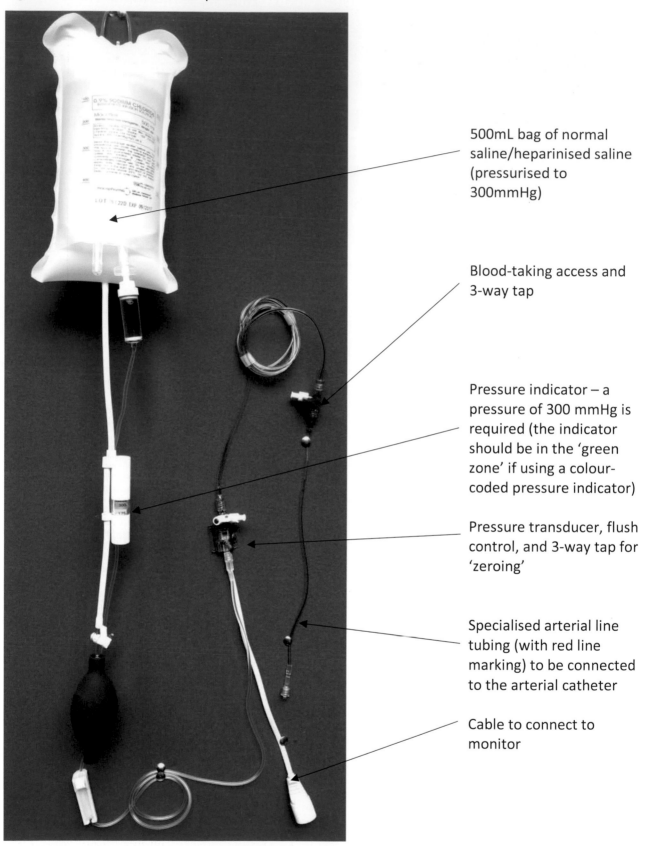

500mL bag of normal saline/heparinised saline (pressurised to 300mmHg)

Blood-taking access and 3-way tap

Pressure indicator – a pressure of 300 mmHg is required (the indicator should be in the 'green zone' if using a colour-coded pressure indicator)

Pressure transducer, flush control, and 3-way tap for 'zeroing'

Specialised arterial line tubing (with red line marking) to be connected to the arterial catheter

Cable to connect to monitor

The arterial waveform

- Reflects the pressure generated in the arteries following ventricular contraction and relaxation giving:
  - Systolic, diastolic and mean arterial pressure measurements
- The dicrotic notch (on the down stroke of the arterial waveform) is caused by the closure of the aortic valve in the heart

Figure 6.3 An example of an arterial line trace

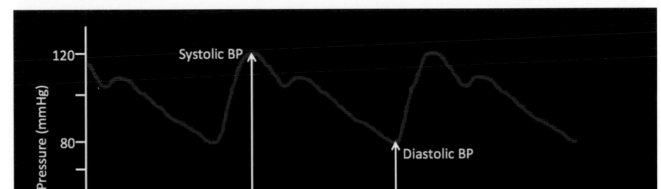

Normal and damped arterial line traces

A normal arterial line trace has 'two peaks' per cardiac cycle and looks a bit like a Scottish mountain range. Damping can be seen when there is a problem within the arterial line system and the line flattens/smooths out (damped trace, sometimes called an 'over-damped' trace) or exaggerates the peak (under-damped trace) of the arterial line trace.

Damping occurs due to anything that prevents the arterial pressure wave from being easily transmitted from the artery, up the column of saline in the arterial line to the pressure transducer, e.g.:

- Air bubbles
- Kinks in the arterial cannula (e.g. flexed wrist with a cannula in the radial artery)
- Blood clots
- Overly compliant tubing (hence you need to use dedicated arterial line tubing which is much stiffer than that used for an intravenous infusion line)
- Port taps being partially opened
- Low pressure in the fluid bag, or empty fluid bag

Under-damping occurs because of excessive vibration within the arterial line system.

A normal arterial line trace (**Figure 6.4**) that is not damped or under-damped, can be said to be optimally damped.

Figure 6.4 A normal ('optimally damped') arterial line trace

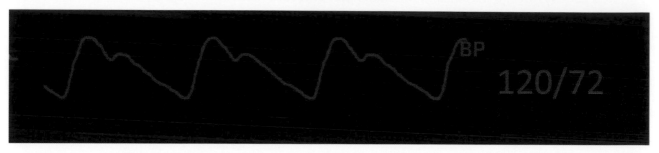

Damped arterial line traces:

A damped arterial line trace will underestimate the systolic blood pressure and overestimate the diastolic blood pressure. If it is not recognised that a trace is damped, an incorrect blood pressure reading will be recorded. A damped trace looks more like rolling hills than mountains.

Figure 6.5 A damped/over-damped arterial trace

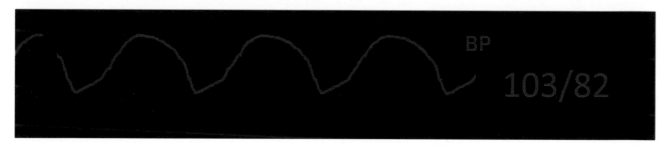

Underdamped arterial line traces:

An under-damped arterial line trace will overestimate the systolic blood pressure. If it is not recognised that a trace is damped an incorrect blood pressure reading will be recorded. An under-damped trace looks like a range of steep Alpine mountains.

Figure 6.6 An underdamped arterial trace

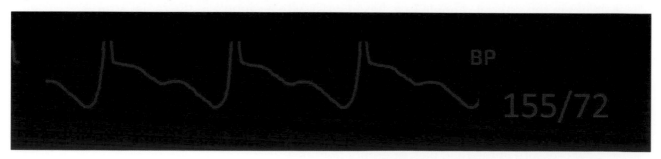

Factors that influence the arterial line reading

- Transducer position - i.e. the transducer is not level with the right atrium (this is the most common cause of significant errors). If the pressure transducer falls to the floor it is not only reading the blood pressure at the level of the heart but also measuring the pressure difference between the heart and the floor – this will lead to an incorrectly high blood pressure reading.
- Insufficient calibration of the transducer (i.e. not regularly 'zeroed')
- Damped or under-damped trace

Management of a woman with an arterial line

- Close monitoring of the woman for signs of complications (e.g. arterial bleeding)
- A 500 mL bag of 0.9% saline/heparinised saline should remain pressurised to 300 mmHg, and the giving set should be changed every 48 hours
- Ensure all connections are secure to prevent bleeding, infection and air emboli
- Document any interventions and/or changes
- Renew dressing as per protocol, or when wet or loose
- Arterial lines should be removed as soon as clinically indicated

Removal of an arterial line

- Check the woman's clotting profile
- Ensure peripheral access (in case of bleeding after removal)
- Aseptic procedure
- Remove dressing
- Slowly remove the catheter whilst applying digital pressure with gauze until bleeding stops (minimum 5 minutes)
- Dress with gauze and clear dressing
- Check the catheter is complete including the tip
- Check the end of the catheter and skin for signs of infection – if concerned send the arterial line for microbiological testing.

Central lines (central venous catheters)

This is a catheter placed in one of the large central veins (superior or inferior vena cava). They usually have three to five ports and provide central venous access for:

- Measurement of central venous pressure (CVP)

- Administration of irritant drugs such as inotropes and amiodarone.
- Parenteral feeding (TPN)
- Obtaining blood for tests (specifically the central venous oxygen saturation)
- Venous access problems
- Long term intravenous access.

Figure 6.7 Three port ('triple lumen') central line

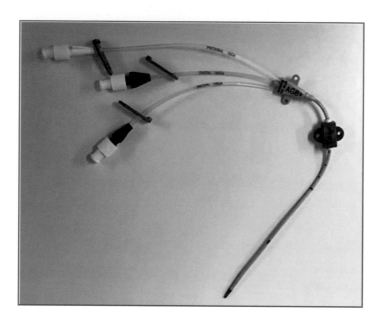

Line insertion

- The lines can be placed into:
  - Neck (internal jugular vein – this is the most common site)
    - The line tip is in the superior vena cava
  - Chest (subclavian vein)
    - The line tip is in the superior vena cava
  - Groin (femoral vein)
    - The line tip is in the inferior vena cava

- Remember to:
  - Explain the procedure to the woman
  - Position the woman slightly head down (for a neck or chest line)
  - Use a full aseptic technique for insertion (i.e. hat, gloves, mask, gown)
  - Have continuous ECG monitoring during insertion

Equipment required for central insertion and monitoring

- Central venous catheter
- Many hospitals have a sterile pre-packed kit containing the necessary disposables
    - 5 mL and 10 mL syringes
    - Sterile gauze
    - Needles for injection
    - 0.9% saline flush solution
    - Sterile drape
    - Suture material (e.g. 2/0 silk on a straight needle)
    - Occlusive transparent dressing
- Chlorhexidine 2% solution or 'snap-stick' for skin preparation
- Ultrasound machine and sterile probe cover
- Sterile gloves, gown and mask
- Local anaesthetic (usually 10 mL 1% lidocaine)
- Transducer set run through from 500 mL 0.9% normal saline/heparinised saline bag
- Pressure bag at 300 mmHg
- Transducer cable
- The operator should be fully 'scrubbed', and wearing a hat, mask, sterile gown and gloves

Potential complications associated with central lines

At insertion	During maintenance	At removal
- Arterial puncture - Pneumothorax - Haemothorax - Haemorrhage - Haematoma - Air embolus - Cardiac arrhythmias - Cardiac tamponade - Incorrect position of catheter tip	- Pneumothorax - Cardiac arrhythmias - Cardiac tamponade - Line infection - Sepsis - Thrombosis	- Haemorrhage - Haematoma - Air embolus - Catheter embolism

Uses of central lines:

- Estimate the circulating blood volume
- Guide fluid administration
- Assist in the assessment of cardiac function and vascular tone
- Aid the assessment of response to treatment, e.g. fluid challenge

However:

- An isolated CVP reading can be misleading
- Trends in CVP are usually more useful than one-off readings
- CVP is often not a reliable marker of left-ventricular filling
- Other parameters e.g. HR, capillary refill, BP and urine output should also be considered

Taking a CVP measurement

- Explain to the woman what you are going to do
- Flush the line to check its patency
- Position the woman supine (if possible) and align the transducer with the fifth intercostal space in the mid-axilla (the surface landmark for the right atrium of the heart).
- Check the CVP trace
- Document the reading and report any changes or abnormalities

The CVP waveform

Figure 6.8 An example of a CVP waveform

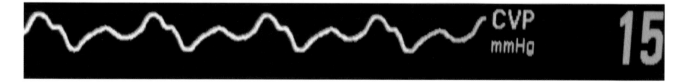

The CVP reflects mean right atrial pressure during the cardiac cycle. A normal CVP reading, measured as described above, is 5–10 mmHg.

- Factors that **increase** CVP readings:
  - Transducer position is below the level of the right atrium – this gives a falsely high CVP reading
  - Hypervolemia
  - Forced exhalation
  - Tension pneumothorax
  - Heart failure

- Pleural effusion
- Decreased cardiac output
- Cardiac tamponade
- Factors that **decrease** CVP readings:
  - Transducer level above the right atrium– this gives a falsely low CVP reading
  - Hypovolemia
  - Deep inhalation

Management of a pregnant or postpartum woman with a CVP line:

- Close monitoring for signs of complications
- Document any interventions, changes and line length at the skin
- Renew dressing as per protocol or when wet or loose
- Label the various ports with drugs/fluids etc.
- If not in use, flush the ports regularly
- The 500 mL bag of 0.9% saline/heparinised saline should remain pressurised to 300 mmHg, and the giving set should be changed every 48 hours
- Ensure all connections are secure to prevent bleeding, infection and air embolus
- CVP lines should be removed when clinically indicated.

Removal of a CVP line:

- Check the woman's clotting profile and medication chart e.g. consideration of timings of last doses of low molecular weight heparin, anti-coagulants etc
- Patient position: supine with a slight head down tilt
- Ensure no drugs are attached and running through the CVP line
- Aseptic procedure
- Remove dressing
- Cut and remove any stitches
- Slowly remove the catheter (if there is resistance then stop and call for assistance)
- Apply pressure with gauze until bleeding stops (minimum 5 minutes)
- Dress with gauze and clear dressing
- Check the catheter is complete including the tip.
- Check the end of the catheter and skin for signs of infection.

Zeroing the transducer lines

Every four hours, both the arterial and CVP pressure transducers should be zeroed, to calibrate them with zero pressure (atmospheric pressure).

- Position woman supine (on their back)
- The head of the bed may be elevated between 0–60°
- Flush the system using the plastic pull flush on the transducer
- Level the transducer, i.e. align the transducer with the fifth intercostal space mid-axilla (level with the right atrium)
- Turn the tap on the port closest to the transducer such that it is 'off' to the woman
- Remove the cap such that the system is 'open to air' (i.e. atmospheric pressure)
- Press zero on the monitor module
- Ensure that zero appears on the monitor screen, then replace the cap and turn the tap so that it is open to the woman.

Troubleshooting invasive pressure monitoring systems

Problem	Solution
Difficulty with zeroing	• Check all equipment and connections between woman and monitor • Ensure all roller-clamps are open • Check the system for air bubbles and blood clots • Check flush bag volume and pressure • Replace transducer, cable, module, arterial cannula
Unable to aspirate cannula	• Check line for kinks • Apply traction to cannula • Gently try to flush manually • Replace arterial line
Falsely high readings	• Incorrect placement of transducer (i.e. placed below level of the heart) • Calibration issues • Under-damped trace • Swapped invasive pressure cables
Falsely low readings	• Incorrect placement of transducer (i.e. placed above level of the heart) • Kinked cannula • Damped trace • Swapped invasive pressure cables
Damped trace	• Check position of transducer • Re-'zero' • Remove kink • Remove air bubbles/ blood clots

Reference

1. AAGBI Safety Guideline: Arterial line blood sampling: preventing hypoglycaemic brain injury. Available from https://www.aagbi.org/sites/default/files/Arterial%20line%20blood%20sampling.pdf. Accessed 8 June 2018.

Section 7: Cardio-respiratory emergencies in pregnant and postpartum women

> **Key learning points**
>
> - Cardio-respiratory diseases are a significant cause of maternal morbidity and mortality
> - The physiological changes of pregnancy can worsen the effects and impact of cardio-respiratory diseases
> - Acquired heart disease such as ischaemic heart disease and aortic dissection can occur in pregnant and postnatal women
> - Investigations and treatments of life-threatening illnesses should not be denied because a woman is pregnant or breastfeeding

Background

During pregnancy changes occur in the mother's body to support the developing fetus; providing warmth, nutrients and oxygen, and removing waste products. These changes in maternal physiology, as outlined below, have the potential to exacerbate pre-existing medical conditions, or trigger new disorders.

Women with pre-existing cardiorespiratory diseases such as asthma, cystic fibrosis, systemic or pulmonary hypertension, congenital heart disease, valvular disease, arrhythmias or other cardiac pathology may find their conditions worsen during pregnancy, compromising the health of both the woman and her unborn baby. In addition, new conditions may manifest during pregnancy such as pre-eclampsia, gestational asthma, acute pulmonary oedema and cardiomyopathy. It is important to note that a significant majority of women who die in pregnancy do so as a result of pre-existing underlying illness.

Normal pregnancy-related cardiovascular changes

Cardiovascular changes start at about 6 weeks' gestation and include:

- *Increased blood volume:*
  - o Blood volume reaches a peak increase of about 45% by 32 weeks' gestation (an extra volume of between 1.2–1.6 L)
  - o The distribution of fluid in the body shifts and by the third trimester there is an increase in both the interstitial (extracellular) fluid and plasma volume.
  - o The increased volume of fluid within the body is partly due to the effects of oestrogen on the renin-angiotensin system (a hormone system that helps regulate sodium balance, fluid volume and blood pressure)
  - o Fetal growth and the birth weight correlate directly with the increase in plasma volume. A reduction in plasma volume is linked to intrauterine growth restriction (IUGR), babies who are small for gestational age (SGA) and pre-eclampsia.

- *Increased red blood cell production:*
  - o This requires an increased consumption of iron meaning the pregnant woman is at risk of iron deficiency.
  - o Despite the increase in red blood cell mass (the pregnant woman has more red blood cells than a non-pregnant woman) the plasma volume increases to a greater degree resulting in a lower haemoglobin concentration than in the non-pregnant state. When this causes anaemia, it is known as the physiological anaemia of pregnancy.

- *Increase in cardiac output:*
  - o Increased stroke volume (the volume of blood pumped from the left ventricle of the heart per beat)
  - o Increased heart rate: the heart rate increases by about 20 beats per minute by 32 weeks' gestation.

- *Blood pressure:*
  - o Initially decreases with the advancing pregnancy until about 20 to 24 weeks' gestation, then begins to rise to pre-pregnancy levels by term.
  - o Systemic vascular resistance (the resistance to blood flow in the circulation) decreases due to vasodilation, reaching about 35% below normal at around 24 weeks' gestation, from when it remains fairly stable.

- *Aortocaval compression:*
  - o Changes in maternal position can alter the cardiac output due to compression of the

inferior vena cava (IVC) by the enlarging uterus, thus reducing return of blood to the heart.

- o Lateral positioning allows near-normal venous return; a supine position however will compress the IVC and reduce cardiac output – this should be avoided.

Summary of terms:

- **Cardiac output**: the volume of blood being pumped by the heart per minute.
- **Stroke volume**: the volume of blood pumped from the left ventricle of the heart with each beat
- **Systemic vascular resistance**: the resistance to flow that must be overcome to push blood through the circulatory system.

Normal pregnancy related pulmonary changes:

- Hormonal changes in pregnancy, particularly related to high levels of progesterone cause a 40% increase in tidal volume (the volume of air that comprises a normal breath). This means that more air passes in and out of the lungs compared to the non-pregnant state and as such, more carbon dioxide is expired leading to lower carbon dioxide levels in the blood ($PaCO_2$).
- An increase in maternal metabolism also results in an increase in oxygen consumption by about 20–30% at term.
- Initially the increased oxygen consumption is matched by an increase in cardiac output. However, as pregnancy progresses, oxygen consumption exceeds the increase in cardiac output.

- **Normal physiological changes during pregnancy have the potential to exacerbate pre-existing cardiorespiratory conditions or may lead to new disorders**
- **Be aware of the physiological changes in pregnancy when assessing an acute illness**

Cardiac disorders in pregnancy:

In the UK, cardiac disease is the leading cause of indirect maternal death, as well as the most frequent cause of maternal death overall. In MBRRACE-UK reports, over 25% of the deaths occurring in pregnancy or postpartum were attributed to a cardiovascular cause (1). The reports identify many circumstances where pregnant or postpartum women had clear symptoms and signs of cardiac disease which were not recognised, often because the diagnosis of heart disease was not considered as a possibility in young pregnant women. Importantly, 77% of the women who died were **not known** to have pre-existing cardiac problems.

It is essential that there is early involvement of senior clinicians from the obstetric and cardiology teams whenever a pregnant or postpartum woman presents with suspected cardiac symptoms.

> **All clinicians should be alert to the possibility of undiagnosed cardiac disease in pregnant women or women who have recently given birth. Staff must also be aware that the normal changes in pregnancy can mimic and mask the symptoms of cardiac conditions, potentially delaying diagnosis.**

Women may have a known history of cardiac disease, including:

- Congenital heart disease
- Ischaemic heart disease
- Pulmonary hypertension
- Severe systemic ventricular dysfunction (as seen in peripartum cardiomyopathy)
- Dilation of the aortic root more than 4 cm (often seen in Marfan's syndrome)
- Severe left-sided obstructive lesions (such as aortic or mitral stenosis).

Chest pain with ECG changes or a new cardiac murmur may help to establish a diagnosis; **however, raised respiratory rate, chest pain, persistent tachycardia and orthopnoea (shortness of breath lying flat) are important signs too. Investigations must not be delayed just because of pregnancy: prompt diagnosis is vital.**

Management of cardio-respiratory emergencies in pregnancy and postpartum:

Immediate management

As with all emergencies, a structured ABCDE approach and an early call for help is key. For all women where cardiorespiratory compromise is suspected, a structured approach starting with a primary survey and secondary should take place (see **Figure 7.1**).

- Call for help

- Supplemental oxygen

- Position:

    o <u>sit-up</u> if there are breathing difficulties or chest pain

    o <u>left lateral</u> if reduced consciousness or hypotensive

- In any cardiorespiratory emergency it is useful to have:

    o baseline observations

    o IV access, routine bloods

    o venous or arterial blood gas

    o 12 lead ECG

- However, obtaining these observations and investigations should not delay calling for medical or obstetric review should the situation require it.

Other considerations:

- Women with cardiorespiratory disease often need to be sat up to improve their breathing. However, do not forget the impact of aortocaval compression if a woman is lying supine, and consider manual displacement of the uterus if necessary

- Warmed fluids and a warming blanket are useful if the woman is hypothermic

- Blood glucose control is important – aim for blood glucose between 4–8 mmol/L

- Thromboprophylaxis – compression stockings, subcutaneous heparin or LMWH

- Stress ulcer prophylaxis – regular proton pump inhibitor (e.g. omeprazole) or H_2-receptor antagonist (e.g. ranitidine)

- May require additional imaging: echo, V/Q scan or CTPA

Figure 7.1 Structured approach to cardio-respiratory emergencies

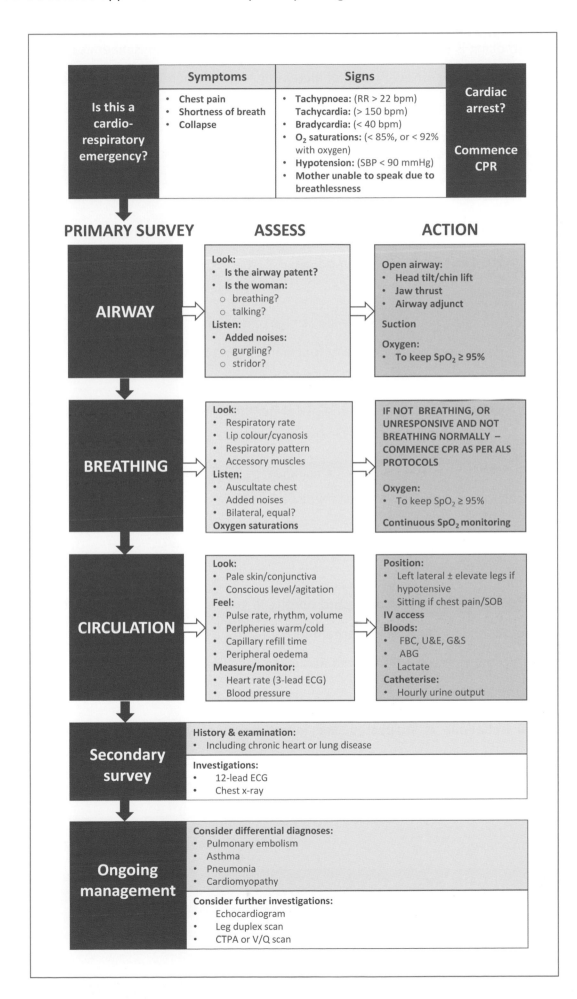

Is this a cardio-respiratory emergency?	Symptoms	Signs	Cardiac arrest? Commence CPR
	• **Chest pain** • **Shortness of breath** • **Collapse**	• **Tachypnoea:** (RR > 22 bpm) • **Tachycardia:** (> 150 bpm) • **Bradycardia:** (< 40 bpm) • **O₂ saturations:** (< 85%, or < 92% with oxygen) • **Hypotension:** (SBP < 90 mmHg) • **Mother unable to speak due to breathlessness**	

PRIMARY SURVEY   **ASSESS**   **ACTION**

AIRWAY	**Look:**
	• **Is the airway patent?**
	• **Is the woman:**
	  o breathing?
	  o talking?
	Listen:
	• **Added noises:**
	  o gurgling?
	  o stridor?
		Open airway:
		• **Head tilt/chin lift**
		• **Jaw thrust**
		• **Airway adjunct**
		
		Suction
		
		Oxygen:
		• **To keep SpO₂ ≥ 95%**

BREATHING	**Look:** • Respiratory rate • Lip colour/cyanosis • Respiratory pattern • Accessory muscles **Listen:** • Auscultate chest • Added noises • Bilateral, equal? **Oxygen saturations**	**IF NOT BREATHING, OR UNRESPONSIVE AND NOT BREATHING NORMALLY – COMMENCE CPR AS PER ALS PROTOCOLS** **Oxygen:** • To keep SpO₂ ≥ 95% **Continuous SpO₂ monitoring**
CIRCULATION	**Look:** • Pale skin/conjunctiva • Conscious level/agitation **Feel:** • Pulse rate, rhythm, volume • Peripheries warm/cold • Capillary refill time • Peripheral oedema **Measure/monitor:** • Heart rate (3-lead ECG) • Blood pressure	**Position:** • Left lateral ± elevate legs if hypotensive • Sitting if chest pain/SOB **IV access** **Bloods:** • FBC, U&E, G&S • ABG • Lactate **Catheterise:** • Hourly urine output

Secondary survey	**History & examination:** • Including chronic heart or lung disease
	Investigations: • 12-lead ECG • Chest x-ray

Ongoing management	**Consider differential diagnoses:** • Pulmonary embolism • Asthma • Pneumonia • Cardiomyopathy
	Consider further investigations: • Echocardiogram • Leg duplex scan • CTPA or V/Q scan

Ischaemic heart disease

In the UK between 2009 and 2014, 34 pregnant women or new mothers died from ischaemic heart disease [1]. Smoking is the single factor most strongly associated with ischaemic heart disease in pregnancy. In pregnancy, for every year of increasing maternal age there is a 20% increase in the risk of myocardial infarction [2].

Box 7.1 Risk factors for ischaemic heart disease

- Obesity
  - 50% of women who died from a cardiac cause in the UK between 2009 and 2014 were overweight or obese
- Increasing age
  - risk of cardiac death is twice as high in women aged 35–39 years
  - risk of cardiac death nearly four times higher in women 40 years or older
- Smoking
  - smokers have 2.5 times the risk of death compared to non-smokers
- Diabetes
- Hypertension
- Family history of premature coronary disease
- Hypercholesterolaemia

With increasing maternal age, smoking and obesity in young women, ischaemic heart disease is likely to remain a major cause of maternal morbidity and death. Both smoking and obesity are preventable. Women should be educated about the specific cardiac risk of pregnancy and which symptoms to report (**Box 7.2**).

If myocardial ischaemia is suspected, the investigation of women in pregnancy or in the postpartum period should be the same as for the general population.

- Physical examination to assess haemodynamic status and elicit signs of any complications
- Serial 12-lead ECGs
- Troponin levels

It is vital that a diagnosis is made in a woman presenting with chest pain.

A negative troponin or V/Q scan should prompt continued investigation until a diagnosis is reached

---

Box 7.2 Chest pain which may be indicative of cardiac ischaemia

- Discomfort developing over minutes in the anterior chest or epigastric area

- Band-like, squeezing, sensation of pressure

- Radiation to the jaw, arms, shoulders

- Radiation into the back

- Associated with breathlessness

- Associated with nausea and/or sweating

- Associated with syncope (fainting)

If the history is consistent with ischaemia, **a normal ECG and/or negative troponin do not exclude the diagnosis** and further investigation should be considered.

The management of suspected acute coronary syndrome is given in **Figure 7.2**.

> **A woman requiring strong analgesia for chest pain must be investigated.**
>
> **Serial 12-lead ECGs should be recorded as soon as possible in a pregnant or postpartum woman presenting with chest pain**

Ergometrine (contained within Syntometrine®) produces vasoconstriction and can cause coronary artery vasospasm and myocardial ischaemia. Ergometrine was a factor associated with the deaths of two women from atherosclerotic coronary disease in the UK between 2009 and 2014 (1). Both women developed chest pain shortly after being given Syntometrine® and both had a cardiac arrest. Severe postpartum haemorrhage may also result in myocardial ischaemia though this is more commonly due to hypovolaemia and inadequate oxygen delivery to the heart muscle. This is best treated using an ABCDE approach, stopping the bleeding and use of blood products as appropriate.

Figure 7.2 The management of suspected acute coronary syndrome

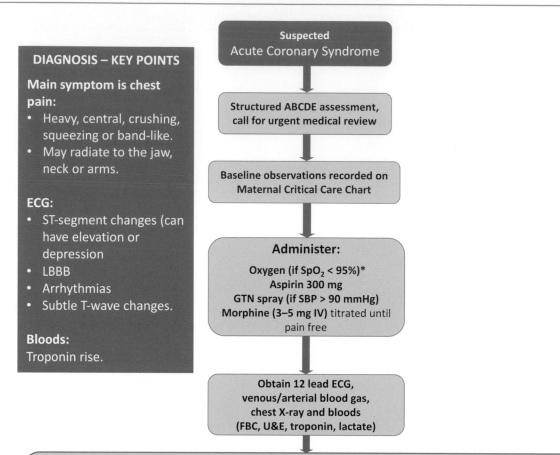

DIAGNOSIS – KEY POINTS

Main symptom is chest pain:
- Heavy, central, crushing, squeezing or band-like.
- May radiate to the jaw, neck or arms.

ECG:
- ST-segment changes (can have elevation or depression
- LBBB
- Arrhythmias
- Subtle T-wave changes.

Bloods:
Troponin rise.

Suspected
Acute Coronary Syndrome

Structured ABCDE assessment, call for urgent medical review

Baseline observations recorded on Maternal Critical Care Chart

Administer:

Oxygen (if SpO$_2$ < 95%)*
Aspirin 300 mg
GTN spray (if SBP > 90 mmHg)
Morphine (3–5 mg IV) titrated until pain free

Obtain 12 lead ECG, venous/arterial blood gas, chest X-ray and bloods (FBC, U&E, troponin, lactate)

From this point onwards, advanced management should be guided by the medical team in collaboration with the senior obstetric team.

If the woman is ante-partum, there should be an appropriate assessment of fetal well-being, and a plan for expediting birth may be necessary.

Advanced

Further investigation and management should be guided by medical personnel.

It may be difficult to confirm the diagnosis from history/examination/ECG alone and therefore instigating treatment may require a careful assessment of risk/benefit.

Treatment of confirmed/suspected acute coronary syndrome involves administration of aspirin 300mg ± further antiplatelet agents (clopidogrel, ticagrelor or prasugrel) depending on local policy.

Definitive management may involve percutaneous coronary intervention which might require transfer to another centre. This is not a risk-free procedure and can carry additional risks in the pregnant or postpartum woman. Early discussion between between the cardiology and obstetric teams is essential in minimising this risk. Also remember that ACS in pregnancy may be due to coronary artery dissection.

*There is increasing evidence that high flow oxygen therapy can increase the size of an infarct and worsen outcome. Oxygen should therefore be titrated to keep SpO$_2$ > 94%.

Aortic dissection

Dissection of the aorta is a rare but frequently fatal event that describes tearing of the wall lining the aorta. Blood pushes through this tear and sits between the layers of the aortic wall. This can be contained with a dissection sac but can result in disruption to arteries arising from the aorta. As such, the presentation of this condition can be varied, but can include chest pain (commonly severe tearing pain and often intra-scapular or going through to the back), change in conscious level or neurological symptoms or pain/ischaemia in one of the limbs.

The majority of aortic dissections in women of childbearing age occur during late pregnancy and the puerperium, time periods that are associated with a 25-fold increased risk of dissection (3). In the UK between 2009 and 2014, 21 women died as a result of an aortic dissection (1). Eight women (42%) had presented in the days before their deaths with symptoms suggestive of significant pathology, such as severe chest and intra-scapular pain, but a diagnosis of aortic dissection was not considered. Five further women (26%) presented acutely unwell with atypical chest or back pain and neurological symptoms including faecal incontinence and leg weakness due to dissection of the entire aorta, but the diagnosis of dissection was delayed or missed.

The commonest mode of death is extension of a dissection of the ascending aorta into the aortic root causing haemopericardium and tamponade. Death rates rise with every hour of delay between the onset of the dissection and control of the haemorrhage in theatre. Aortic dissection that extends into the arterial tree can cause neurovascular symptoms as well as pulseless limbs and severe localising chest and back pain.

> The classic symptoms of aortic dissection are severe tearing chest pain radiating to the back. Pain severe enough for a mother to leave her baby at home in the night to attend the Emergency Department requires a diagnosis: co-existing anxiety and musculoskeletal pain should not be accepted as the cause.
>
> The diagnosis of aortic dissection should be considered in women who present with neurological symptoms as well as chest and back pain, as the condition may be missed if only neurological causes are considered.

Ventricular dysfunction and pulmonary oedema

There are many causes of ventricular dysfunction in pregnancy, including cardiomyopathy (i.e. structural heart muscle disease). Cardiomyopathies can be acquired or inherited, may be primary or secondary and principally fall into dilated, hypertrophic or restrictive types. Peripartum cardiomyopathy is a form of dilated cardiomyopathy that typically occurs in late pregnancy or postpartum. Whatever the aetiology, a poorly functioning ventricle may be unable to provide the increased cardiac output required in pregnancy, resulting in pulmonary oedema and an increased risk of arrhythmia.

Acute pulmonary oedema may also develop as a result of a single, significant cardiovascular event, such as pre-eclampsia causing an extremely high blood pressure, or cardiogenic shock as a complication of myocardial ischemia. Pulmonary oedema may also result from inappropriate intravenous fluid administration.

Symptoms of pulmonary oedema include:	Signs include:
<ul><li>Sudden onset breathlessness</li><li>Agitation</li><li>Coughing</li><li>Orthopnoea</li></ul>	<ul><li>Tachypnoea</li><li>Tachycardia</li><li>Fine inspiratory crackles (and possibly wheeze) on auscultation</li><li>Decreased oxygen saturation</li><li>Changes in the chest x-ray</li></ul>

Pink frothy sputum is very suggestive of pulmonary oedema and should be investigated and treated accordingly.

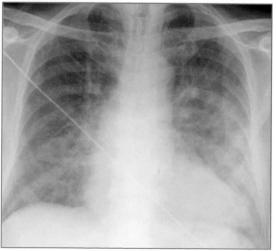

Figure 7.3 Chest x-ray demonstrating pulmonary oedema

There were no maternal deaths due to inappropriate fluid management (pulmonary oedema and renal failure) in the UK between 2003 and 2014 (1), which demonstrates clear improvement in the awareness and management of pulmonary oedema in pregnancy and the postnatal period.

Figure 7.4 The management of suspected pulmonary oedem

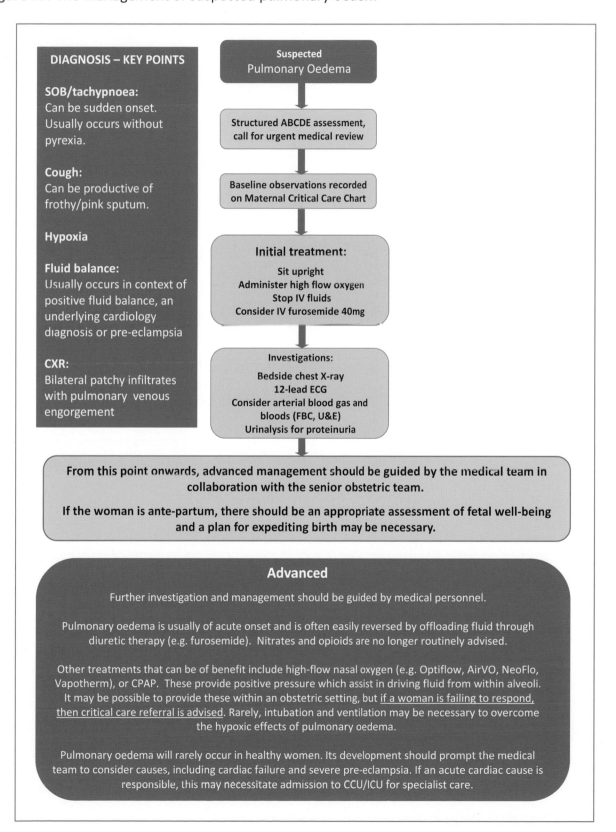

Respiratory disorders

Pulmonary embolism:

> **Risk factors and predisposing factors for pulmonary oedema include:**
>
> - Pre-existing cardiac disease
>   - Hypertension
>   - Ischemic heart disease
>   - Arrhythmias
> - Specific diseases in pregnancy
>   - Pre-eclampsia
>   - Sepsis
>   - Cardiomyopathy
>   - Pulmonary embolism
> - Pharmacologic agents
>   - Beta-adrenergic
>   - Tocolytic agents
>   - Corticosteroids
>   - Illicit drug use
> - Fluid overload from fluid administration (usually intravenous but can be secondary to large volumes of oral fluid intake)
>   - Positive fluid balance of > 2,000 mL
>   - IV fluid administration is frequently a major preventable risk factor
> - Multiple pregnancies (eg, twins, triplets).

Venous thromboembolic disease remains one of the most common causes of direct maternal death and therefore being able to promptly recognise, investigate and treat this condition is of paramount importance in reducing avoidable maternal deaths.

Pulmonary embolism, a blood clot in one or more of the pulmonary arteries, is classically caused by the embolisation of a deep vein thrombosis (DVT) from the leg or pelvic veins. Risk factors for DVT are given by Virchow's triad: venous stasis, endothelial injury and hypercoagulability. Pregnancy increases at least two of these risks, whilst critical illness in pregnancy predisposes to all three. All women should undergo a documented venous thromboembolism (VTE) risk assessment in early pregnancy; this must be repeated if the woman is admitted to hospital and should be reassessed after birth. This is especially important in women rendered immobile and pro-inflammatory by critical illness.

Symptoms of pulmonary embolus include:
- Sudden onset breathlessness
- Pleuritic chest pain; i.e. sharp, stabbing pain that is worse on deep breathing or coughing
- Cough ± haemoptysis (coughing up blood)
- Shortness of breath
- Collapse

Signs include:
- Tachypnoea
- Tachycardia
- Decreased oxygen saturation
- Auscultation of the chest is usually normal, although a pleural 'rub' may be heard
- Raised jugular venous pressure may be noted
- Deep vein thrombosis may be evidenced by tender leg swelling ± discolouration

A CXR and 12-lead ECG should be performed. CXR is usually normal in pulmonary embolus. 12-lead ECG will usually show a sinus tachycardia, and may show S1, Q3, T3 (deep S-wave in lead I, Q-waves and T-wave inversion in lead III) as signs of right-heart strain; however, a *small* Q-wave and T-wave inversion can be normal variants in pregnancy. An arterial blood gas may be useful to confirm hypoxaemia.

If a PE is suspected on clinical examination, diagnosis may be confirmed by investigating for DVT by duplex ultrasound of the deep leg veins. However, if there is no clinical evidence of DVT, the diagnosis can be made by ventilation/perfusion (V/Q) scan or by CT pulmonary angiography (CTPA); liaise with your local radiologist to determine the most appropriate investigation (4). An urgent bedside echocardiogram (if available) may be useful to diagnose right-heart strain in massive, life-threatening pulmonary embolus.

The initial management of pulmonary embolus is shown in **Figure 7.5**

Figure 7.5 The management of suspected pulmonary embolus (PE)

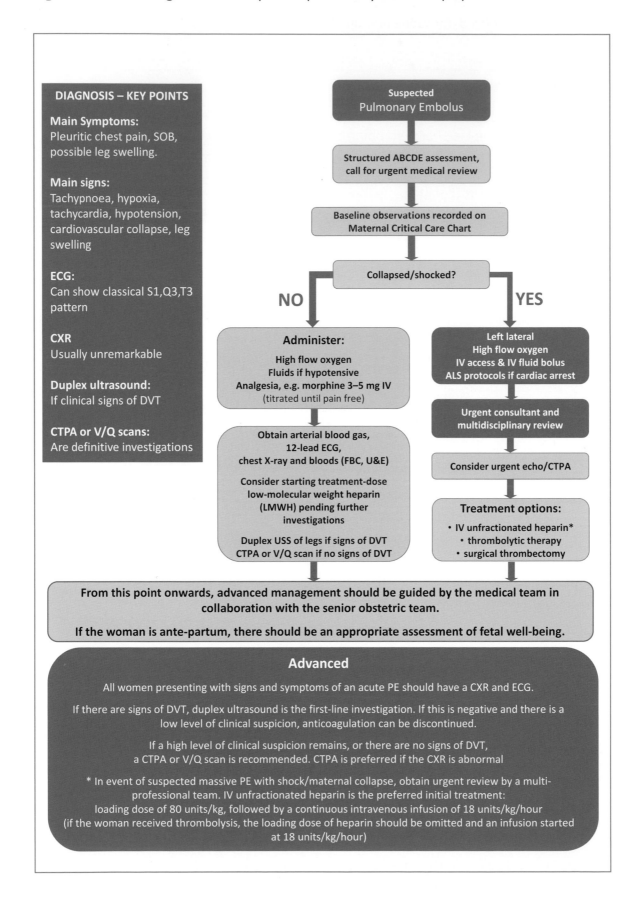

The mainstay of treatment is stabilisation using an ABCDE approach, and by anticoagulation

using treatment-dose low-molecular weight heparin (LMWH; e.g. enoxaparin (Clexane®), tinzaparin). This should be started immediately if there is a high index of suspicion of pulmonary embolus, unless there are significant contraindications.

Definitive treatment will require anticoagulation for a period of at least 3 months. This can carry significant risk in the pregnant or postnatal woman and therefore, the decision to continue treatment in the absence of a definite diagnosis of pulmonary embolus needs to be balanced against the individual woman's risks and benefits.

> **'Women should not be denied relevant investigations or treatments for life-threatening conditions, simply because they are pregnant or breastfeeding.' (2)**

Asthma:

- During pregnancy about one third of women with pre-existing asthma show an improvement in their condition, about one third get worse, and one third have no change in their symptoms
- Aggravating factors that may worsen asthma include:
  - gastro-oesophageal disease
  - changes in chest wall conformation
  - an increase in upper respiratory tract infections.

Figure 7.6 The initial management of suspected acute severe asthma

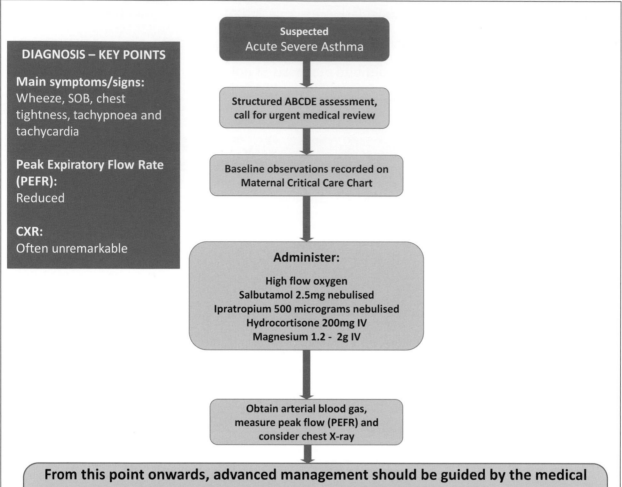

DIAGNOSIS – KEY POINTS

Main symptoms/signs:
Wheeze, SOB, chest tightness, tachypnoea and tachycardia

Peak Expiratory Flow Rate (PEFR):
Reduced

CXR:
Often unremarkable

Suspected
Acute Severe Asthma

Structured ABCDE assessment, call for urgent medical review

Baseline observations recorded on Maternal Critical Care Chart

Administer:

High flow oxygen
Salbutamol 2.5mg nebulised
Ipratropium 500 micrograms nebulised
Hydrocortisone 200mg IV
Magnesium 1.2 - 2g IV

Obtain arterial blood gas, measure peak flow (PEFR) and consider chest X-ray

From this point onwards, advanced management should be guided by the medical team in collaboration with the senior obstetric team.

If the woman is ante-partum, there should be an appropriate assessment of fetal well-being.

Advanced

If acute severe asthma is suspected, an urgent medical review should be requested and treatment should be instituted. As part of a medical assessment it is helpful to classify the severity of acute asthma:

Severity	PEFR*	Other features
Acute	50–75%	No features of severe asthma
Severe	33–50%	Unable to complete sentences in one breath
Life-threatening	<33%	SpO_2 < 92% / PaO_2 < 8 kPa on air, silent chest, cyanosis, altered conscious level, hypotension, arrhythmias
Near-fatal		Rising $PaCO_2$ / requiring mechanical ventilation

Life-threatening or near-fatal asthma both warrant urgent referral to intensive care.

* Repeat assessment of PEFR is helpful in assessing response to treatment.

- During pregnancy, a woman with asthma has an increased risk of pre-eclampsia, excessive vomiting, gestational diabetes, low birth weight, and premature birth.
- As with non-pregnant asthmatics, pregnant women are encouraged to take steps to control asthma symptoms and follow an asthma action plan:
  - avoid triggers such as smoking
  - continue to take medications effectively
  - seek early intervention if symptoms do not improve with self-management.

The initial management of acute severe asthma is given in **Figure 7.6**.

Cystic Fibrosis (CF):

- Premature birth is the most common complication for pregnant women with cystic fibrosis, with approximately 24% of women with severe CF delivering preterm.
- Cystic fibrosis in pregnancy requires regular monitoring of the woman's respiratory function and coordinated multidisciplinary management by a specialist team.

References

1. Knight M, Nair M, Tuffnell D, Kenyon S, Shakespeare J, Brocklehurst P, et al. Saving Lives, Improving Mothers' Care. Knight M, Nair M, Tuffnell D, Kenyon S, Shakespeare J, Brocklehurst P, on behalf on MBRRACE-UK. Oxford National Perinatal Epidemiology Unit, University of Oxford. 2016.

2. Bush N, Nelson-Piercy C, Spark P, Kurinczuk JJ, Brocklehurst P, Knight M, et al. Myocardial infarction in pregnancy and postpartum in the UK. Eur J Prev Cardiolog. 2012 Dec 20;20(1):12–20.

3. Nasiell J, Lindqvist PG. Aortic dissection in pregnancy: the incidence of a life-threatening disease. Eur J Obstet Gynecol Reprod Biol. 2010 Mar;149(1):120–1.

4. Thromboembolic Disease in Pregnancy and the Puerperium: Acute Management. Green Top Guideline No 37b. RCOG. April 2015. Available from https://www.rcog.org.uk/globalassets/documents/guidelines/gtg-37b.pdf. Accessed on 2nd December 2017.

Section 8: Neurological emergencies in pregnant and postpartum women

---

> **Key learning points**
> - New-onset neurological symptoms require investigation
> - Headache of sudden onset or with an abnormal neurological examination are red-flag signs
> - Any change in consciousness is a sign of critical illness and should be acted upon
> - Prolonged or frequent seizures may be due to a neurological condition, rather than eclampsia

Background

Deaths from neurological causes remain a leading cause of indirect maternal death in the UK (1). Benign headaches are common during pregnancy, but staff should be aware that a headache may be a sign of a potentially life-threatening neurological emergency.

Common causes of headaches in pregnant/postnatal women include:

- Simple/tension headache (usually bilateral)
- Migraine:
  - usually unilateral ± aura (often visual), nausea and vomiting, photophobia
  - the woman will usually have a history of identical migraines
- Drug-related (usually vasodilators, e.g. nifedipine)
- Post-dural-puncture headache:
  - in women who have had recent epidural or spinal anesthesia
  - classically postural in nature (worse on sitting/standing, relieved by lying down), bilateral (frontal or occipital) and severe)

The physiological changes of pregnancy increase the risk of a woman having an acute neurological condition:

- Pregnancy is a hypercoagulable state with increases in clotting factors, especially fibrinogen and factor VIII. This increases the risk of cerebral thrombosis and ischaemic stroke

- Raised blood volume, cardiac output and changes in vascular tone may contribute to the potential for intracerebral haemorrhage, e.g. cerebral aneurysm rupture. The risk of intracerebral haemorrhage is especially high in severe pre-eclampsia, owing to the disruption to the vascular endothelium

RED FLAG FEATURES OF HEADACHE
- Sudden onset
- Associated with neck stiffness
- 'Worst headache ever'
- Abnormal signs on neurological examination

An acute neurological deterioration during pregnancy may be due to an exacerbation of a pre-existing condition or a new presentation of a neurological condition. Common causes of neurological emergencies in pregnancy are outlined below.

Exacerbation of a pre-existing condition	New condition
Epilepsy Other seizure disorders Multiple sclerosis	Brain tumour Stroke: • Intracerebral haemorrhage • Ischaemic stroke Cerebral venous thrombosis Infections: • Meningitis • Encephalitis Posterior reversible encephalopathy syndrome (PRES)

Clinical Diagnosis

A neurological emergency may present with:

- An altered level of consciousness
- Seizures
- Headache
- Severe hypertension
- Limb or facial weakness
- Sensory changes
- Speech impairment
- Visual disturbance

Figure 8.1 Structured approach to neurological emergencies

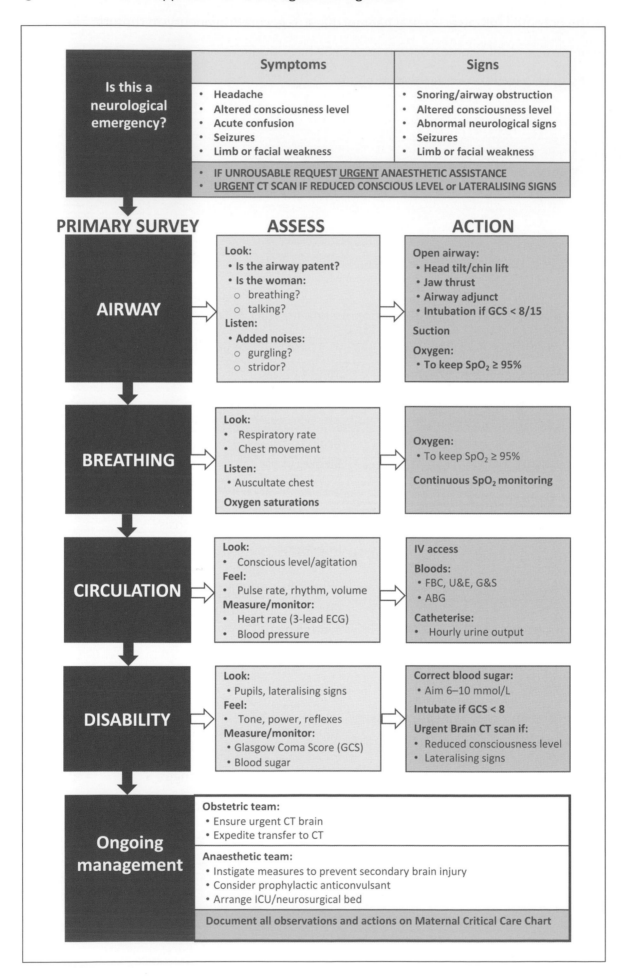

	Symptoms	Signs
Is this a neurological emergency?	• Headache • Altered consciousness level • Acute confusion • Seizures • Limb or facial weakness	• Snoring/airway obstruction • Altered consciousness level • Abnormal neurological signs • Seizures • Limb or facial weakness
	• IF UNROUSABLE REQUEST <u>URGENT</u> ANAESTHETIC ASSISTANCE • <u>URGENT</u> CT SCAN IF REDUCED CONSCIOUS LEVEL or LATERALISING SIGNS	

PRIMARY SURVEY **ASSESS** **ACTION**

AIRWAY

Look:
• Is the airway patent?
• Is the woman:
  o breathing?
  o talking?
Listen:
• Added noises:
  o gurgling?
  o stridor?

Open airway:
• Head tilt/chin lift
• Jaw thrust
• Airway adjunct
• Intubation if GCS < 8/15
Suction
Oxygen:
• To keep SpO$_2$ ≥ 95%

BREATHING

Look:
• Respiratory rate
• Chest movement
Listen:
• Auscultate chest
Oxygen saturations

Oxygen:
• To keep SpO$_2$ ≥ 95%
Continuous SpO$_2$ monitoring

CIRCULATION

Look:
• Conscious level/agitation
Feel:
• Pulse rate, rhythm, volume
Measure/monitor:
• Heart rate (3-lead ECG)
• Blood pressure

IV access
Bloods:
• FBC, U&E, G&S
• ABG
Catheterise:
• Hourly urine output

DISABILITY

Look:
• Pupils, lateralising signs
Feel:
• Tone, power, reflexes
Measure/monitor:
• Glasgow Coma Score (GCS)
• Blood sugar

Correct blood sugar:
• Aim 6–10 mmol/L
Intubate if GCS < 8
Urgent Brain CT scan if:
• Reduced consciousness level
• Lateralising signs

Ongoing management

Obstetric team:
• Ensure urgent CT brain
• Expedite transfer to CT

Anaesthetic team:
• Instigate measures to prevent secondary brain injury
• Consider prophylactic anticonvulsant
• Arrange ICU/neurosurgical bed

Document all observations and actions on Maternal Critical Care Chart

Signs and symptoms can mimic minor common ailments such as headaches, but staff should be aware of the red flag features listed above. Similarly, it is worth noting that agitation and restlessness may be a sign of an underlying problem in women with hypertension (2).

Any women with new onset symptoms in keeping with a neurological disorder should be comprehensively assessed and should have consideration of further investigation. Baseline observations should be taken, and bloods should be sent to exclude electrolyte or clotting abnormalities.

If a neurological emergency is suspected in a pregnant, or postpartum women, a standardised approach to management is advised. This should begin with calling for help, and an ABCDE approach to assessment and management. An algorithm for the structured approach to neurological emergencies is given in **Figure 8.1**.

Beyond these initial tests, a significant number of acute neurological disorders seen in pregnancy can be investigated and confirmed/excluded with radiological imaging such as CT or MRI scans of the head.

Specific Neurological Disorders

Hypertensive disorders:

Hypertensive disorders are the second most common cause of maternal death worldwide (3). Between 2011 and 2013, six women in the UK died as a direct result of pre-eclampsia or eclampsia (4). In addition, one in 400 000 women giving birth in the UK die from pregnancy-related hypertensive disorders (5). Whilst the incidence of maternal death attributable to pre-eclampsia and eclampsia in the UK has decreased significantly over the past five years (currently 0.13/100 000 maternities) (1), it is imperative that we continue to recognise and promptly treat these conditions to aim to further reduce deaths and morbidity from hypertensive disorders of pregnancy.

The single largest major failing in clinical care remains inadequate treatment of systolic hypertension resulting in intracranial haemorrhage. It is crucial to remember that severe hypertension (systolic blood pressure above 160 mmHg) is an obstetric emergency and must be treated urgently to prevent maternal mortality and morbidity (6).

> **Keep blood pressure in all women below 150/100 mmHg, with urgent treatment to achieve this in women with severe systolic hypertension (SBP ≥ 160 mmHg).**
>
> **Do not administer ergometrine alone or in combination with another drug (e.g. Syntometrine®) for management of the third stage of labour in the presence of known maternal hypertension, or if maternal blood pressure has not been taken during labour**
>
> **Whilst intubation may occasionally be required for airway control, maternal stabilisation and blood pressure control is vital prior to intubation of hypertensive women to minimise maternal risk.**

Neuroimaging should be performed urgently in any woman with hypertension or pre-eclampsia who has focal neurology, or who has not recovered from a seizure.

Clinical examination of women with neurological symptoms and hypertension should include a full neurological examination, including fundoscopy. There should be awareness of agitation and restlessness as a sign of an underlying problem. Neuroimaging should be considered early in women with atypical eclampsia. This includes those with multiple fits, those with only mildly increased blood pressure or proteinuria, and those who do not become fully conscious within an hour of their fit. Whilst most of these women will have normal neurological anatomy, in some, treatable intracranial pathology may be diagnosed.

- Neurological examination, including fundoscopy, is mandatory in all women with new onset headaches or headache with atypical symptoms (4).
- Neurological examination including assessment for neck stiffness is mandatory in all new onset headaches or headache with atypical features, particularly focal symptoms.
- Pregnancy should not alter the standard of care for women with stroke. All women with stroke, pregnant or not, should be admitted to a Hyper-acute Stroke Unit.
- Neither pregnancy, caesarean section birth nor the immediate postpartum state are absolute contraindications to thrombolysis (intravenous or intra-arterial), clot retrieval or craniectomy (7).

Cerebrovascular events:

Cerebrovascular events (CVEs) include ischaemic and haemorrhagic stroke, subdural haematoma, aneurysm rupture and cerebral venous sinus thrombosis. Subdural haemorrhage and cerebral venous sinus thrombosis are well-recognised complications of pregnancy. Both should also be included in the differential diagnosis of persistent headache after inadvertent dural puncture ('dural tap') or after post-dural-puncture headache (PDPH). Any woman who suffers an inadvertent dural puncture or post-dural-puncture headache must be notified to her GP and routine follow-up arranged.

A cerebrovascular event can present with any of the symptoms associated with neurological disorders. As such, it may be more difficult to make a specific diagnosis on clinical examination alone.

> **Signs that make a cerebrovascular event more likely include:**
>
> - sudden onset
> - unilateral weakness
> - changes in sensation
> - speech impairment
> - drop in conscious level
> - pupillary asymmetry

An ABCDE approach, and early radiological investigation, are crucial to confirming a diagnosis and guiding ongoing management.

If conscious level is significantly affected due to an intracerebral event (i.e. GCS ≤ 8/15, or unresponsive/responds to pain on AVPU), it is likely that the airway will need to be secured. Should the woman require transfer to another hospital for neurosurgical intervention, it should be remembered that inter-hospital transfer of a woman with a reduced level of consciousness requires appropriate medical (usually anaesthetic) involvement (8).

Cerebral vein thrombosis:

Thrombosis of the cerebral veins that drain the brain (e.g. cortical veins and cerebral sinuses) is uncommon but is more likely in pregnant/postnatal women owing to the hypercoagulable state of pregnancy. Its presentation is variable, depending on the area of the brain affected, but can consist of:

- severe headache
- seizures
- reduced consciousness/coma
- dizziness

- nausea and vomiting
- abnormal neurological examination

Performing a CT of the brain alone is usually insufficient to diagnose cerebral venous thrombosis; therefore, if there is a high index of clinical suspicion, CT venography or MR (magnetic resonance) venography should be requested.

Initial treatment involves stabilising ABCDE, with specific treatment options being guided by local expertise; this may involve anticoagulation, and occasionally endovascular thrombolysis or surgical thrombectomy.

Epilepsy:

Epilepsy is the most common serious neurological disease affecting pregnant/postnatal women in high-income countries; one percent of the UK population is affected, and 23% of people with epilepsy are women of child-bearing age (9). Epilepsy related mortality is increased with pregnancy (10), and epilepsy remains an important indirect cause of maternal death.

Whilst seizures in a pregnant or postpartum woman with epilepsy are most likely to be due to epilepsy, it should be kept in mind that a new condition can co-exist. It is crucial to rule out the development of eclampsia or any other neurological disorder, rather than assuming that a seizure in an epileptic pregnant woman is definitely due to epilepsy.

Most epileptic seizures in pregnant women are likely to be isolated, short-lived and self-terminating. Status epilepticus is a life-threatening neurological emergency which occurs when a seizure lasts for longer than five minutes, or when two seizures occur in quick succession without full neurological recovery in between. Rapid assessment and treatment are essential to protect the airway, prevent hypoxia, and prevent brain injury or fetal compromise.

Figure 8.2 Management of suspected status epilepticus

DIAGNOSIS – KEY POINTS

Epileptic seizures include:
- absence seizures
- tonic-clonic seizures

Associated symptoms and signs:
- changes in vision
- changes in smell
- urinary incontinence
- tongue biting

Status epilepticus definition:
- Any epileptic seizure lasting more than 5 minutes

Or:
- Recurrent seizures without full neurological recovery in between

Suspected Status epilepticus

↓

Structured ABCDE assessment, call for urgent medical review

↓

**Position in left lateral
Head-tilt, chin-lift
High flow oxygen**

↓

If a seizure has not stopped within 5 minutes administer:

Lorazepam 4 mg IV

**If no IV access give either:
Diazepam 10 mg PR, or
Midazolam 10 mg buccal**

↓

**Obtain baseline observations
Consider ABG, urinalysis + lab bloods**

↓

From this point onwards, advanced management should be guided by the medical team in collaboration with the senior obstetric team.

If the woman is ante-partum, there should be an appropriate assessment of fetal well-being.

Advanced

It can be difficult to determine whether seizures in the second half of pregnancy are due to epilepsy or eclampsia. If doubt exists, treatment for eclampsia must be commenced alongside management of epilepsy until definitive examination and investigations can exclude eclampsia as a cause.

Seizures during labour should be terminated as soon as possible to minimise maternal and fetal hypoxia and to reduce the development of maternal and fetal acidosis.

If a seizure is not terminated by an initial dose of benzodiazepine (IV lorazepam, PR diazepam or buccal midazolam) then a repeat dose may be given after 10–15 minutes.

If repeated doses of benzodiazepine do not stop seizure activity, a loading dose of phenytoin should be given intravenously (dose = 15mg/kg – commonly around 1000mg). If administration of phenytoin fails to stop seizure activity, consideration must be given to induction of general anaesthesia with the possibility of requiring urgent/emergent delivery of the baby.

Assessment of Conscious Level

AVPU:

The AVPU scale, as described in Chapter 2, is the quickest way to give an assessment of conscious level. It is easy to perform, reliable and can help guide ongoing management and need for airway support.

A	Alert
V	Responds to **Voice**
P	Responds to **Painful** stimulus (corresponds to GCS $\leq$ 8)
U	**Unresponsive**

Glasgow Coma Score (GCS):

This is a standardised assessment of conscious level comprising three sections (eyes, verbal and motor) and allows a more in-depth assessment than AVPU.

To perform a GCS, go through each section systematically (eyes, motor, verbal), scoring the patient's best response, then combine to give a total score.

Glasgow Coma Score:

Eyes:
4	Opens eyes spontaneously
3	Opens eyes in response to voice
2	Opens eyes in response to painful stimuli
1	Does not open eyes

Verbal:
5	Oriented, converses normally
4	Confused, disoriented
3	Utters inappropriate words
2	Incomprehensible sounds
1	Makes no sounds

Motor:
6	Obeys commands
5	Localises to painful stimuli
4	Flexion/withdrawal to painful stimuli
3	Abnormal flexion to painful stimuli
2	Extension to painful stimuli
1	Makes no movements

Both individual elements and the total score are important, so for example record as:

- GCS is 9 = E2 V4 M3.

The lowest possible score is a GCS of 3 (E1 V1 M1), as the lowest score in each category is 1.

Pupil response:

Pupils should be of equal size and should respond similarly to light and accommodation by constriction (PERLA = pupils equal and reactive to light and accommodation).

Unequal pupil responses should prompt further enquiry. An abnormally dilated pupil on one side may be caused by localised raised intracranial pressure (e.g. following an intracerebral haemorrhage), which stretches the oculomotor (III) nerve. A constricted pupil on one side may be caused by a Horner's syndrome, e.g. from a unilateral high spinal anaesthetic block.

Ongoing management, and prevention of secondary brain injury:

Primary brain injury is the initial neurological insult. Secondary brain injury is injury that occurs after this, e.g. due to:

- further neurological insult (e.g. ongoing intracerebral haemorrhage, uncontrolled seizures)
- cerebral oedema
- raised intracranial pressure
- hypoxia
- infection

Secondary brain injury is often preventable through appropriate clinical management, using an ABCDE approach:

- Monitor vital signs every 15 to 60 minutes and record findings on a maternal critical care chart
- Intubate and ventilate women with reduced conscious level to prevent raised CO_2 and hypoxia
- Maintain cerebral perfusion pressure (CPP)
  - cerebral perfusion pressure is the mean arterial pressure minus intracranial pressure (ICP). Patients with raised intracranial pressure will need a higher mean arterial blood pressure to ensure adequate brain perfusion (typically aim for MAP of 80 mmHg)
- Control seizures
- Normoglycaemia
  - aim for blood glucose between 6–10 mmol/L
- Re-consider CT or MRI if not already performed
  - neuroimaging should be performed urgently in any woman with hypertension

or pre-eclampsia who has focal neurology or who has not recovered from a seizure

- Consider early liaison with the ICU team particularly if the woman has required intubation.

Other considerations:

- Thromboprophylaxis:
  - compression stockings, subcutaneous heparin or LMWH
  - note that medical prophylaxis must be considered against the risk of intracerebral bleeding
- Stress ulcer prophylaxis:
  - regular PPI (e.g. omeprazole) or H_2-receptor antagonist (e.g. ranitidine)
- Paracetamol for persistent pyrexia

> **Early detection of neurological conditions can prevent secondary brain injuries**
>
> **Neurological disease in pregnancy can be life threatening and is associated with significant morbidity and mortality**

References

1. Knight M, Nair M, Tuffnell D, Shakespeare J, Kenyon S, Kurinczuk JJ (Eds.) on behalf of MBRRACE-UK. Saving Lives, Improving Mothers' Care - Lessons learned to inform maternity care from the UK and Ireland Confidential Enquiries into Maternal Deaths and Morbidity 2013–15. Oxford: National Perinatal Epidemiology Unit, University of Oxford 2017.

2. National Collaborating Centre for Women's and Children's Health. *Hypertension in Pregnancy: the management of hypertensive disorders during pregnancy.* NICE Clinical Guideline. London: Royal College of Obstetricians and Gynaecologists; 2011.

3. Kassebaum et al. Global, regional, and national levels and causes of maternal mortality during 1990-2013: a systematic analysis for the Global Burden of Disease Study 2013. *Lancet* 2014;384:980-1004.

4. Knight M, Tuffnell D, Kenyon S, Shakespeare J, Gray R, Kurinczuk JJ (Eds.) on behalf of MBRRACE-UK. Saving Lives, Improving Mothers' Care - Surveillance of maternal deaths in the UK 2011-13 and lessons learned to inform maternity care from the UK and Ireland Confidential Enquiries

into Maternal Deaths and Morbidity 2009-13. Oxford: National Perinatal Epidemiology Unit, University of Oxford 2015.

5.   Knight M; UKOSS. Eclampsia in the United Kingdom 2005. Br J Obstet Gynaecol 2007; 114: 1072-8.

6.   Douglas KA, Redman CW. Eclampsia in the United Kingdom. *Br Med J* 1994; 309: 1395-400.

7.   Knight M, Kenyon S, Brocklehurst P, Neilson J, Shakespeare J, Kurinczuk JJ (Eds.) on behalf of MBRRACE- UK. Saving Lives, Improving Mothers' Care - Lessons learned to inform future maternity care from the UK and Ireland Confidential Enquiries into Maternal Deaths and Morbidity 2009–12. Oxford: National Perinatal Epidemiology Unit, University of Oxford 2014.

8.   AAGBI Safety Guideline: Interhospital Transfer. Available from
     https://www.aagbi.org/sites/default/files/interhospital09.pdf. Accessed 9 June 2018.

9.   Epilepsy prevalence, incidence and other statistics: Joint Epilepsy Council of the UK and Ireland. Available from
     http://www.epilepsyscotland.org.uk/pdf/Joint_Epilepsy_Council_Prevalence_and_Inci
     dence_September_11_(3).pdf. Accessed 9 June 2018

10. Adab N, Kini U, Vinten J, Ayres J, Baker G, Clayton-Smith J, Coyle H, Fryer A, Gorry J, Gregg J, Mawer G, Nicolaides P, Pickering L, Tunnicliffe L, Chadwick DW. The longer-term outcome of children born to mothers with epilepsy. J Neurol Neurosurg Psychiatry. 2004 Nov; 75(11): 1575-83.

Section 9: Sepsis and the critically ill pregnant or postpartum woman

---

Key learning points

- Recognise that pregnant and postpartum women are at risk of sepsis
- Understand the importance of Sepsis Six
- Recognise that Sepsis Six is the launchpad for the full sepsis resuscitation care bundle
- Discussion with ICU is required when a woman is unresponsive to Sepsis Six or where lactate is >4 mmol/L

What is sepsis?

Sepsis is a life-threatening condition that arises when the body's response to an infection injures its own tissues and organs (1). The source of the infection may be found in a particular body region (e.g. chorioamnionitis) or may be widespread in the bloodstream, resulting in septicaemia. Sepsis is a medical emergency because it can result in an interruption to the supply of oxygen and nutrients to vital organs such as the brain, heart, liver, kidneys, lungs and intestines, resulting in acidosis, organ failure and death. General sepsis management is covered in more detail in **Module 8** of the PROMPT 3 Course Manual (Third Edition).

> **Genital tract infection is a common source of sepsis in pregnant and postpartum women, and is a leading cause of maternal mortality**

The immune changes associated with normal pregnancy mean that pregnant women are susceptible to developing sepsis (2). Pregnant or postpartum women are usually relatively young and fit and can often withstand the effects of sepsis until it is extensive. Therefore, pregnant women and new mothers can often appear relatively well, sometimes up until their point of collapse. Women with medical co-morbidities, or those who have undergone surgical interventions, are at increased risk of sepsis; however, previously fit and healthy women with normal pregnancies and straightforward vaginal births also continue to die from sepsis. Sepsis remains a leading cause of maternal mortality and morbidity (2).

Potential causes of maternal sepsis	
Pregnancy related	**Non-pregnancy related**
<ul><li>Chorioamnionitis following:<ul><li>Retained products of conception</li><li>Prolonged ruptured membranes</li><li>Amniocentesis or CVS</li></ul></li><li>Postoperative causes:<ul><li>Caesarean birth</li><li>Operative vaginal delivery</li><li>Cervical suture</li><li>Haematoma</li></ul></li><li>Breast abscess or mastitis</li><li>Urinary tract infection</li></ul>	<ul><li>Pneumonia</li><li>Influenza</li><li>Meningitis</li><li>Appendicitis (which may present atypically)</li><li>Pyelonephritis (more common in pregnancy)</li><li>Cholecystitis</li><li>Bowel perforation (more common with inflammatory bowel disease)</li><li>Cellulitis</li></ul>

Identifying pregnant and postpartum women with sepsis

Sepsis manifests in a variable combination of clinical symptoms and signs, and the diagnosis is supported by laboratory findings. The onset of life-threatening sepsis in pregnancy or the puerperium can be insidious or may show extremely rapid clinical deterioration, particularly when it is the result of streptococcal infection. It is therefore essential that all staff, including community midwives, maternity care assistants, health visitors, emergency department staff and general practitioners are aware of the signs and symptoms of sepsis to avoid unnecessary delays in referral to hospital and treatment (3).

Signs and symptoms of maternal sepsis	
Symptoms	**Signs**
• Fever	• Tachypnoea
• Diarrhoea	• Hypotension
• Vomiting	• Tachycardia
• Abdominal pain	• Pyrexia (> 38 °C) or hypothermia (< 36 °C)
• Sore throat	• Rash (scarlet patches over generalised redness or petechial)
• Cough (especially productive)	• Low oxygen saturations (< 95% on air)
• Offensive vaginal discharge	• Poor peripheral perfusion (capillary refill > 2 seconds)
• Wound infection	• Pallor
• Breast tenderness or focal swelling	• Clamminess
	• Anxiousness, confusion, feeling of 'impending doom'
	• Altered mental state
	• Mottled skin
	• Low urine output (< 0.5mL/kg/hour)
	• MOEWS: 1 or more RED scores

Signs to look out for in the pregnant or postpartum woman:

▪ *Temperature:*

   o Pyrexia is common, but a normal temperature does not exclude sepsis. Paracetamol and other analgesics may mask pyrexia and this should be considered when assessing women who are unwell.

   o Hypothermia (Temperature < 36 °C) is a significant finding that may indicate severe infection and should not be ignored.

   o Swinging pyrexia and failure to respond to broad-spectrum intravenous antibiotics is suggestive of a persistent focus of infection or abscess.

▪ *Heart rate:*

   o Persistent tachycardia > 100 bpm is an important sign which may indicate serious underlying disease and should be fully investigated.

- *White cells:*
  - Leucopenia (< 4 x 10^9 white blood cells/L) is a significant finding that may indicate severe infection.
  - Leucocytosis (> 12 x 10^9 white blood cells/L) may be a significant finding, but can also be elevated as a normal finding in the peripartum phase.

- *Diarrhoea* is a common and important symptom of pelvic sepsis. Diarrhoea and/or vomiting in a woman with any evidence of sepsis can be a serious sign and an indication for commencing immediate broad-spectrum intravenous antibiotic therapy.

- *Severe lower abdominal pain and severe 'after-pains' that require frequent analgesia* or do not respond to the usual analgesia are also common and important symptoms of pelvic sepsis. In some cases, very severe lower abdominal pain may be the result of the action of bacterial toxins on the bowel wall. On rare occasions overwhelming streptococcal infection can present with generalised abdominal pain in the absence of pyrexia and tachycardia

- *An abnormal or absent fetal heart beat* with or without placental abruption may be the result of sepsis

- *Elevated C-reactive protein (CRP)* is an early marker of infection (especially bacterial) which should initiate regular observations of vital signs, initiate investigations to locate a source of infection, and consider whether antibiotic treatment is indicated

Bacterial and viral throat swabs should be taken when a pregnant woman or a mother who has recently given birth presents to healthcare professionals with a sore throat or respiratory symptoms. There should be a low threshold for antibiotic treatment.

Infection must be suspected and actively ruled out when a pregnant or recently delivered woman has:
  - A low or high temperature
  - Persistent bleeding
  - Abdominal pain, especially if the pain is constant and severe
  - A history of prolonged rupture of membranes or chorioamnionitis

Investigations include:

- *Immediate Blood Tests*
    - Blood cultures
    - Lactate

- *Other Blood Tests*
    - FBC
    - Urea & electrolytes and glucose (± capillary blood glucose)
    - CRP
    - Clotting
    - Liver function tests

- *Microbiology*
    - Swabs: e.g. throat, vaginal, viral
    - Mid-stream urine
    - Other relevant: sputum, breast milk, stool, etc.
    - If infection suspected during labour or birth (offensive liquor, baby born in poor condition) swabs should be taken from vagina, placenta, and baby (ear and skin) and the neonatal team should be informed. Ask the neonatal team if swabs from the baby have grown any organisms.

- *Radiology/Imaging*
    - Pelvic ultrasound to check for retained products of conception
    - Other as indicated – chest x-ray, renal ultrasound etc.

Septic shock:

This is a subset of sepsis in which the woman has significant cardiovascular and organ dysfunction, in which she remains hypotensive despite fluid resuscitation. Mortality in patients with septic shock can be as high as 40% (1), and so prompt treatment with IV antibiotics and fluid therapy – and early referral to intensive care – are vital.

Septic shock
Sepsis in which, after adequate fluid resuscitation: ■ Vasopressors are required to maintain MAP ≥ 65 mmHg   <u>and</u> ■ Lactate > 2 mmol/L

Septic shock can be difficult to recognise. A collapsed mother with sepsis may exhibit all the signs and symptoms of hypovolaemia, but if there is no improvement in the serum lactate 15 minutes after a 500 mL crystalloid bolus, then septic shock should be considered and the woman referred to intensive care for possible vasopressor support (3).

Management

> **Early recognition + early communication**
> **=**
> **Early treatment and lives saved**

Figures 9.1 and 9.2 outline the identification, risk stratification and immediate treatment for pregnant or postpartum women presenting with possible sepsis. **If sepsis is suspected, call for help and institute the 'SEPSIS SIX' bundle within 1 hour**.

Use of the 'Sepsis Six' is only the first stage of management and each measure is described in more detail in the PROMPT Course Manual (Third edition). Organ failure and mortality are directly linked to ongoing untreated hypotension and shock. 'Sepsis Six' should be used as the platform for early escalation of care if required (3,4).

Sepsis Six ensures that the most urgent, life-saving treatments are given in a timely fashion in septic women. However, it is unlikely to be sufficient on its own to reverse sepsis in the most severe cases.

Figure 9.1 Risk assessment tool for suspected maternal sepsis

Risk Assessment & Action for Suspected Maternal Sepsis
(adapted from UK Sepsis Trust Inpatient Maternal Sepsis Tool - 2016)

PROMPT
Practical Obstetric Multi-Professional Training

1. **Has MEOWS been triggered?**
2. **Does the woman look unwell?**
3. **Is fetal heart rate ≥ 160 bpm?**
4. **Could this woman have an infection?***
   Common infections include:
   - Chorioamnionitis/endometritis
   - Urinary Tract Infection
   - Wound infection
   - Influenza/pneumonia
   - Mastitis/breast abscess

Affix Patient ID

If YES to any of the above, complete risk assessment

High Risk criteria
(tick all those that are appropriate)

- Respiratory rate ≥ 25 ☐
- SpO2 < 92% ☐
- Heart rate > 130 ☐
- Systolic BP ≤ 90 ☐
- Altered mental status/ Responds only to voice, pain or unresponsive ☐
- Blood Lactate ≥ 2.0* ☐
- Non-blancing rash/mottled/ cyanotic ☐
- Urine < 0.5 ml/kg/hr ☐
- No urine for 18 hrs ☐

If ONE criteria is present:

Commence 'Sepsis Six' NOW

- **Immediate obstetric review ST3 or higher** (transfer to Obstetric Unit if in community)
- **Inform Consultant Obstetrician & Consultant Anaesthetist**
- **Commence Maternal Critical Care Chart**
- **Commence 'High Risk of Maternal Sepsis' Proforma**

Moderate Risk criteria
(tick all those that are appropriate)

- Respiratory rate 21–24 ☐
- Heart rate 100 –129 ☐
- Systolic BP 91 –100 ☐
- Temperature < 36 °C ☐
- No urine output for 12–18 hours ☐
- Fetal heart > 160bpm/Non-reassuring CTG ☐
- Prolonged SRM ☐
- Recent invasive procedure ☐
- Bleeding/wound infection/vaginal discharge/abdominal pain ☐
- Close contact with Group A Strep ☐
- Relatives concerned about mental/ functional status ☐
- Diabetes/ gestational diabetes/ immuno-suppressed ☐

If TWO criteria are present (also consider if only ONE criteria):

Send bloods:
FBC, lactate, CRP, LFTs, clotting
OBSTETRIC REVIEW (ST3 or higher) within one hour
Consider 'Sepsis Six'

Review Bloods: If lactate > 2 or Acute Kidney Injury present, follow HIGH Risk Pathway

Low Risk criteria
(tick all those that are appropriate)

- Respiratory rate ≤ 20 ☐
- Heart rate < 100 ☐
- Systolic BP > 100 ☐
- Normal mental status ☐
- Temperature: 36 – 37.3 °C ☐
- Looks well ☐
- Normal CTG ☐
- Normal urine output ☐

If ALL criteria are present:

LOW RISK OF SEPSIS

Review & monitor for improvement or deterioration

Consider obstetric needs & full clinical picture

* Lactate measurement may be transiently elevated during & immediately after normal labour & birth. If unsure, repeat sample.

Completed by:
Name: Designation: Time:
Signature: Date:

Figure 9.2 Maternal Sepsis Six documentation pro forma (adapted from UK Sepsis Trust)

PROMPT
Practical Obstetric Multi-Professional Training ®

High risk of Maternal Sepsis Proforma
(adapted from the UK Sepsis Trust
Inpatient Maternal Sepsis Tool - 2016)

Affix Patient ID

CALL FOR HELP and complete ALL 'SEPSIS SIX' ACTIONS within ONE HOUR	Time zero:	
Action	**Time completed & initials**	**Reason not done/ variance/comments**
1. Administer 100% OXYGEN o 15 L/min via non-rebreathe mask o Aim to keep saturations > 94%		
2. Take BLOOD CULTURES *(but do not delay administering antibiotics)* o Also consider sputum/urine/HVS/throat swab/breast milk sample/ wound swab/stool sample etc		
3. Take bloods – CHECK SERUM LACTATE o If venous lactate raised, recheck with arterial sample o Discuss with critical care if lactate ≥ 4mmol/L o Continue to check serial serum lactates to monitor response to treatment		
4. Give IV BROAD SPECTRUM ANTIBIOTICS (as Trust protocol) o Administer ASAP, consider allergies o Aim to take blood culture first but do not delay antibiotics if culture bottles not available		
5. Give IV FLUID THERAPY o If lactate > 2mmol/L give 500mL stat o If hypotensive or lactate ≥ 4mmol/L can repeat boluses up to 30 mL/kg (e.g. 2 L for a 70 kg woman) o Extreme caution if woman has pre-eclampsia: discuss with anaesthetist		
6. Accurate MEASUREMENT OF URINE OUTPUT o Urinary catheter & hourly measurement o Document fluid balance record		

If after 'Sepsis Six': systolic BP remains < 90mmHg, level of consciousness remains altered, respiratory rate > 25, lactate not reducing (or was previously > 4mmol/L), refer IMMEDIATELY to Critical Care Team

Also consider:
o If antenatal – monitor fetal heart rate/commence CTG
o Remove the source of infection, e.g. retained products, expedite birth
o Refer to Critical Care Team

Document actions taken:

Maternal Sepsis requires multi-professional team input from: (tick staff contacted)

- Midwife coordinator ☐
- Senior/Consultant obstetrician ☐
- Senior obstetric anaesthetist ☐

- Microbiologist ☐
- Intensive/critical care team ☐

Sepsis Six

1. **Give high flow oxygen** via non-rebreather mask at 15 L/min

2. **Take blood cultures**

   - consider sputum/urine/HVS/throat swab/breast milk sample/wound swab/stool sample etc.

3. **Check serum lactate** and take bloods

   - FBC/U&E/LFTs/clotting/CRP/blood glucose

   - consider group & save

4. **Give IV broad spectrum antibiotics** immediately

   - do not delay in order to obtain culture samples

   - do not wait for microbiology results

   - risk of mortality increases 8% for every hour delay in starting antibiotics in septic shock.

5. **Give IV fluids** (e.g. Hartmann's solution) in 500 mL boluses.

   - this can be repeated up to 30 mL/kg

   - extreme caution in severe pre-eclampsia

6. **Accurate measurement of urine output** via urinary catheter on an hourly chart.

If women do not respond to the Sepsis Six, then liaise with the critical care team. It is likely that the woman will need more intensive treatment along the lines of the Surviving Sepsis Care Bundle (see below) (5). This involves a number of actions to be completed within the first three hours, and others to be completed within six hours of presentation to medical care. Most of the actions are already achieved by the Sepsis Six, so attention can then be given to maintaining mean arterial pressure (MAP) ≥ 65 mmHg using vasopressors and assessing the response to ongoing treatment. Whilst administering vasopressors may ultimately require Level 3 ICU care, they can usually be started by an anaesthetist on labour ward.

In one study of non-pregnant patients in a UK hospital diagnosed with sepsis, the patients with the best outcomes were those who received both Sepsis Six <u>and</u> the Surviving Sepsis Care Bundle (4).

Surviving Sepsis Care Bundle (5)

To be completed within 1st hour of presentation:

- Measure lactate level. Re-measure if initial lactate is >2 mmol/L

- Obtain blood cultures (ideally before administering antibiotics)

- Administer broad-spectrum antibiotics

- Begin rapid administration of 30 mL/kg crystalloid for hypotension or lactate $\geq$ 4 mmol/L

- Give vasopressors to maintain MAP $\geq$ 65 mmHg if hypotensive during/after fluid resuscitation

Other considerations:

- Commence observations on a maternal critical care chart

- If antenatal – remember fetal monitoring

- If possible, remove source of infection as applicable e.g. retained products, deliver baby

- Remember care bundles for critical illness:

  - Blood glucose control: aim for blood glucose 6–10 mmol/L

  - Thromboprophylaxis: compression stockings, intermittent pneumatic compression devices, low molecular weight heparin

  - Stress ulcer prophylaxis: regular PPI (e.g. omeprazole) or H_2-receptor antagonist (e.g. ranitidine)

  - Paracetamol for persistent pyrexia

A multi-professional team input is required from

- Midwife coordinator

- Senior obstetrician

- Senior obstetric anaesthetist

- Microbiology

- Intensive care/critical care team

Recognising when a septic pregnant or postpartum woman requires ICU:

When might ICU be needed?
- *Unresponsive to Sepsis Six:*
    - Fluid (up to 30 mL/kg) and IV antibiotics have been administered but:
        - the woman remains hypotensive (SBP < 90 mmHg)
        - the lactate does not reduce
        - consciousness level does not return to normal
        - respiratory rate > 25
    - Vasopressors (e.g. phenylephrine, metaraminol, ephedrine, noradrenaline) may be required from an anaesthetist to maintain MAP ≥ 65 mmHg
- *Lactate > 4.0 mmol/L:*
    - This suggests severe tissue/organ impairment
- *Respiratory failure:*
    - respiratory distress despite oxygen administration
    - low saturations ± PaO_2 on arterial blood gas whilst on high-flow oxygen
- *Uncontrolled agitation:*
    - often caused by hypoxia
- *Acute renal failure:*
    - low or no urine output, raising urea and creatinine
    - may need temporary renal replacement therapy
- *Severe acidaemia:*
    - pH < 7.20
    - this is usually accompanied by a raised lactate

Transferring a critically ill woman to ICU:
- Inform the midwife coordinator that transfer is required so that any available help can be allocated to you.
- You will need help and support with the transfer, including an anesthetist
- Keep monitoring for any deterioration in condition until on ICU.
- Continue ongoing resuscitation and treatment until handing over care.
- Organise transport, equipment (monitoring, oxygen), drugs, detailed notes.
- Make sure ICU are aware of any specific obstetric needs, including support and care to encourage bonding with her baby, if the woman is postnatal.
- Make sure relatives are well informed and have the relevant phone numbers/ directions to ICU.

All transfers are associated with the risk of destabilisation and deterioration and there is a requirement for specialised personnel and equipment. Transfers need to be timely, coordinated, smooth and well-planned. For more information please refer to **Section 1**.

References

1.   Singer M, Deutschman CS, Seymour CW, Shankar-Hari M, Annane D, Bauer M, et al. The Third International Consensus Definitions for Sepsis and Septic Shock (Sepsis-3). JAMA. 2016 Feb 23;315(8):801–10.

2.   Knight M, Kenyon S, Brocklehurst P, Neilson J, Shakespeare J, Kurinczuk JJ, on behalf of MBRRACE-UK. Saving Lives, Improving Mothers' Care. Oxford National Perinatal Epidemiology Unit, University of Oxford. 2014.

3.   Sepsis: recognition, diagnosis and early management. National Institute for Health and Care Excellence. 2017 Dec 2:1–50. Available from https://www.nice.org.uk/guidance/ng51/resources/sepsis-recognition-diagnosis-and-early-management-pdf-1837508256709. Accessed 2nd December 2017.

4.   Daniels R, Nutbeam T, McNamara G, Galvin C. The sepsis six and the severe sepsis resuscitation bundle: a prospective observational cohort study. Emergency Medicine Journal. 2011 May 19;28(6):507–12.

5.   Levy MM, Evans LE, Rhodes A. The Surviving Sepsis Campaign Bundle: 2018 Update. *Crit Care Med.* 2018;997 - 1000